Guided Bone Regeneration in Implant Dentistry

Guided Bone Regeneration in Implant Dentistry

Edited by

Daniel Buser, DDS, PD Dr Med Dent
Associate Professor
Department of Oral Surgery
School of Dental Medicine
University of Berne
Berne, Switzerland

Christer Dahlin, DDS, PhD
Associate Professor
The Brånemark Clinic
Public Dental Health Service
University of Göteborg
Göteborg, Sweden
Department of Oral and Maxillofacial Surgery
Norra Alvsborgs Länssjukhus NÄL
Trollhättan, Sweden

Robert K. Schenk, MD, Prof Dr Med
Professor Emeritus of Anatomy
Institute of Pathophysiology
University of Berne
Berne, Switzerland

quintessence
books

Quintessence Publishing Co, Inc
Chicago, Berlin, London, Tokyo, Moscow, Prague, Sofia, and Warsaw

Library of Congress Cataloging-in-Publication Data

Guided bone regeneration in implant dentistry / edited by Daniel
  Buser, Christer Dahlin, Robert K. Schenk.
     p. cm.
  Includes bibliographical references and index.
  ISBN 0-86715-249-4
  1. Endosseous dental implants. 2. Guided bone regeneration.
I. Buser, Daniel. II. Dahlin, Christer. III. Schenk, Robert K.
  [DNLM: 1. Guided Tissue Regeneration. 2. Dental Implantation,
Endosseous—methods. 3. Bone Regeneration. WU 240 G946 1994]
RK667.I45G84 1994
617.6'9—dc20
DNLM/DLC
for Library of Congress   94-242
                                          CIP

quinte∫∫ence
book∫

Editor: Lori A. Bateman
Designer: Jennifer A. Sabella
Production Manager: Timothy M. Robbins

Composition: Midwest Technical Publications, St Louis, MO
Printing and binding: Everbest Printing Co, Ltd, Hong Kong
Printed in Hong Kong

Contents

Dedicated to the pioneers of
guided bone regeneration:

L.A. Hurley
C.A.L. Bassett
P.J. Boyne
T.P. Rüedi
T. Karring
S. Nyman

Contributors

Jeanne Ambruster
W.L. Gore & Associates, Inc
Flagstaff, Arizona

William Becker, DDS, MSD
Private Practice
Tucson, Arizona
Associate Professor
Department of Periodontics
University of Texas at Houston
School of Dentistry
Houston, Texas

Burton E. Becker, DDS
Private Practice
Tucson, Arizona
Associate Professor
Department of Periodontics
University of Texas at Houston
School of Dentistry
Houston, Texas

Urs C. Belser, DDS, Prof Dr Med Dent
Professor and Chairman
Department of Fixed Prosthetics and Occlusion
University of Geneva
Geneva, Switzerland

Hermann Berthold, Prof Dr Med, Dr Med Dent
Professor and Chairman
Department of Oral Surgery
School of Dental Medicine
University of Berne
Berne, Switzerland

Daniel Buser, DDS, PD Dr Med Dent
Associate Professor
Department of Oral Surgery
School of Dental Medicine
University of Berne
Berne, Switzerland

Christer Dahlin, DDS, PhD
Associate Professor
The Brånemark Clinic
Public Dental Health Service
University of Göteborg
Göteborg, Sweden
Department of Oral and Maxillofacial Surgery
Norra Alvsborgs Länssjukhus NÄL
Trollhättan, Sweden

Karl Dula, DDS, Dr Med Dent
Assistant Professor
Department of Oral Surgery
School of Dental Medicine
University of Berne
Berne, Switzerland

Ross Hardwick, MS
W.L. Gore & Associates, Inc
Flagstaff, Arizona

Hans-Peter Hirt, DDS, Dr Med Dent
Assistant Professor
Department of Oral Surgery
School of Dental Medicine
University of Berne
Berne, Switzerland

Ole T. Jensen, DDS, MS
Assistant Clinical Professor
Department of Oral and Maxillofacial Surgery
University of Colorado
School of Dentistry
Denver, Colorado

Sascha A. Jovanovic, Drs, MS
Section of Periodontics
University of California at Los Angeles
School of Dentistry
Los Angeles, California

Raquel Sanchez
W.L. Gore & Associates, Inc
Flagstaff, Arizona

Todd V. Scantlebury
W.L. Gore & Associates, Inc
Flagstaff, Arizona

Robert K. Schenk, MD, Prof Dr Med
Professor Emeritus of Anatomy
Institute of Pathophysiology
University of Berne
Berne, Switzerland

Nancy Whitley
W.L. Gore & Associates, Inc
Flagstaff, Arizona

Foreword

As this century approaches its close, we find ourselves being flooded by an incredible amount of information daily. Each minute detail of every war, catastrophe, and major sporting event taking place anywhere on earth is painstakingly reported by radio, television, newspapers, and thousands of journals. Our information pool continues to expand exponentially as we in the sciences research, publish, read, research, publish, ... , and as an older human being I ask myself, *Where will this all lead in the next millennium?* One can be assured that much of this information will regulate itself, and that the natural selection process—as it has existed since the creation of earth—will continue to function. Clearly, "everything has its time," as the Bible states so prudently. The dinosaurs had their time, and so will it once be said that amalgam has had its time, too.

In dentistry, implantology currently is in "its time." It is not surprising that new methods are constantly being looked for by the dental profession to improve its various procedures and make them even safer and more predictably successful. Other than the discovery of the phenomenon of osseointegration more than 20 years ago, the concept of *Guided Bone Regeneration* (GBR) represents the most important progress in implant dentistry in the past years. Not long ago, patients with local bone defects often had to be contraindicated for implant treatment. The concept of GBR has drastically changed this unsatisfactory condition and revolutionized implant treatment planning. In this book, the GBR concept—also referred to as *the Membrane Technique*—is portrayed by the best qualified authors from biologic, histologic, and surgical points of view. It is the first time that original information on this topic is presented in a textbook format. This book will undoubtedly receive great attention by the dental profession and will aid in the predictable and successful treatment of implant patients with local alveolar bone deficiencies.

André Schroeder, Dr Med Dent, Dr HC
Professor Emeritus, University of Berne

Preface

The use of barrier membranes for the regeneration of bone defects has significantly changed implant dentistry in the past 5 years. This principle, often called *Guided Bone Regeneration (GBR or GBR technique)*, was first described in 1959 by Hurley et al for the treatment of experimental spinal fusion. In the 1960s, the research teams of Bassett and Boyne tested microporous cellulose acetate laboratory filters (Millipore) for the healing of cortical defects in long bones and for osseous facial reconstruction, respectively. The authors used these filters to establish a suitable environment for osteogenesis by excluding fibrous connective tissue cells from bone defects. However, these pioneering studies did not immediately lead to a broad clinical application of barrier membrane techniques in patients. The clinical potential of the membrane technique was recognized by the research team of Karring and Nyman, who systematically examined barrier membranes in various experimental and clinical studies for periodontal regeneration in the early 1980s. These studies established the basis of a completely new treatment approach in periodontal therapy.

In the late 1980s, barrier membrane techniques were again investigated for bone regeneration in experimental studies. Based on promising results in these studies, clinical testing of membranes began in implant patients in 1988. Five years of intensive experimental and clinical work followed. At this time it seemed appropriate to analyze the current status of "Guided Bone Regeneration in Implant Dentistry," and the idea for the present textbook was borne.

This book is written for the clinician with interest and experience in implant dentistry. The book is structured in two sections focusing on basic science and clinical applications of GBR. As an introduction to the topic of the book, Chapter 1 discusses the current status of implant dentistry. Emphasis is given to anatomic, surgical, and esthetic considerations in the placement of dental implants that satisfy the two major demands of implant patients: long-term function and esthetics.

Chapter 2 deals with basic science aspects of GBR and presents the original experimental studies carried out at the University of Göteborg in the mid-1980s. Chapter 3 covers the biologic basis of bone regeneration. The excellent histology utilizing nondecalcified sections is based on more than 30 years of experience in experimental orthopedic research and conveys the details of bone regeneration in general. Histologic sections of a recently published experimental study demonstrate beautifully the pattern of bone regeneration that occurs underneath e-PTFE membranes in particular. Finally, Chapter 4 describes the design criteria for barrier membranes—such as aspects of biocompatibility, barrier function, and space maintenance—and how these biomaterial considerations affect clinical performance. These three chapters covering the basics of GBR are essential for the reader's understanding of the biologic and biomaterial background of this exciting new technique, knowledge that is crucial for the use of barrier membranes in patients.

In the clinical section of the book, Chapters 5 through 8, procedures associated with different indications of the GBR technique are presented in detail. Each chapter deals with specific indications and describes the criteria for patient selection, the step-by-step surgical procedure, and aspects of postoperative treatment. Emphasis is given to incision technique and flap design; the handling, placement, and stabilization of barrier membranes; the combination of membranes with autogenous bone grafts as a membrane supporting device and osteoconductive scaffold; as well as aspects of wound closure. The clinical results of the GBR technique in numerous patients are critically evaluated and discussed. The four clinical chapters of the book reflect the current clinical status of GBR in implant dentistry; they discuss not only the potential, but also the limitations of this technique in clinical practice.

The editors thank the contributors for their effort and time; they all agreed to participate in this project without hesitation and with great enthusiasm. It has been a very intensive but satisfying experience to collaborate with colleagues of such quality.

CHAPTER ONE

Anatomic, Surgical, and Esthetic Considerations in Implant Dentistry

Daniel Buser
Urs C. Belser

Based on fundamental experimental studies performed by the research teams of Professor P.-I. Brånemark from the University of Göteborg, Sweden, and Professor A. Schroeder from the University of Berne, Switzerland, the use of dental implants has become a scientifically accepted treatment concept in dentistry to replace lost or missing teeth in fully and partially edentulous patients. This breakthrough in implant dentistry was initiated by the discovery that dental implants made of commercially pure titanium can be anchored in the jawbone with direct bone contact. In a landmark paper published in 1969,[1] Brånemark et al described this phenomenon for submerged titanium implants from a clinical point of view and with decalcified histologic sections (the implants had to be removed before sectioning). Seven years later, Schroeder et al[2] provided the first true histologic evidence of direct bone-to-implant contact for nonsubmerged titanium implants using nondecalcified histologic sections with the titanium implants still present in the specimens (Fig 1-1). Later, these authors created the terms *osseointegration*[3] and *functional ankylosis*[4,5] to describe this phenomenon. In the past 10 years, the terms osseointegration and osseointegrated implants have been widely used in the literature and will be used herein.

An osseointegrated implant is characterized in light microscopic analysis by a direct apposition of bone to the titanium surface without evidence of a separating connective tissue layer between the bone and the implant (Fig 1-2). Hereby, the bone has all characteristics of living bone, such as osteocytes or blood vessels, close to the implant surface. Osseointegration has also been documented in scanning electron microscopic (SEM) studies (Fig 1-3)[4,5] as well as in a transmission electron microscopic (TEM) study (Figs 1-4a and b).[6]

To achieve an osseointegrated titanium implant with high predictability, the implant *(1)* must be inserted with a low-trauma surgical technique, avoiding overheating of the bone during preparation of a precise recipient site; *(2)* must be placed with initial stability; and *(3)* should not be functionally loaded during the healing period of 3 to 6 months. When these clinical guidelines are followed, successful osseointegration will occur predictably for nonsubmerged titanium implants (one-stage procedure) as well as for submerged titanium implants (two-stage procedure), as has been demonstrated in comparative experimental studies.[7,8]

The best-documented two-stage implant system is the Brånemark System (Nobelpharma AB, Gothenburg, Sweden), whereas the most prominent one-stage system using nonsubmerged titanium implants with a titanium plasma-sprayed (TPS) surface is the ITI System (Institut Straumann, Waldenburg, Switzerland). The basic characteristics, indications, and clinical procedures of both implant systems have been described in detail in textbooks written by Brånemark et al[9] and Schroeder et al.[10,11]

The long-term documentation of osseointegrated implants was first reported by Adell et al[12,13] in a retrospective clinical study treating fully edentulous patients with Brånemark implants. The authors reported estimated implant survival rates of 86% in the mandible and 78% in the maxilla at 15 years.[13] Data published from prospective studies on fully edentulous patients by Zarb et al[14,15] have confirmed these results. Similar results of retrospective studies have also been reported for nonsubmerged ITI implants placed in fully edentulous patients by Babbush et al,[16] ten Bruggenkate et al,[17] and Krekeler et al.[18]

In the mid-1980s, clinical investigators started to focus more on the treatment of partially edentulous patients in order to expand indications for osseointegrated implants. Although related 10-year data are still lacking for any implant system, encouraging results with ITI implants were found in a prospective study on partially edentulous patients at the University of Berne. Applying strict criteria for success, the examination up to 5 years demonstrated success rates above 95%.[19-21] Mean success rates above 90% have also been reported for Brånemark implants in a prospective study by Zarb and Schmitt.[22,23] Recently, 5-year results with success rates above 90%, applying life table analysis, have also been presented for the IMZ system (Interpore International, Irvine, CA) for fully and partially edentulous patients.[24]

Encouraging treatment results in patients with standard indications have, in the past 5 to 10 years, led to increasing interest in the use of dental implants in "borderline" indications, such as recipient sites with insufficient bone volume, recipient sites close to specific anatomic structures (mandibular nerve, maxillary sinus, etc), extraction sockets, and esthetically demanding sites.

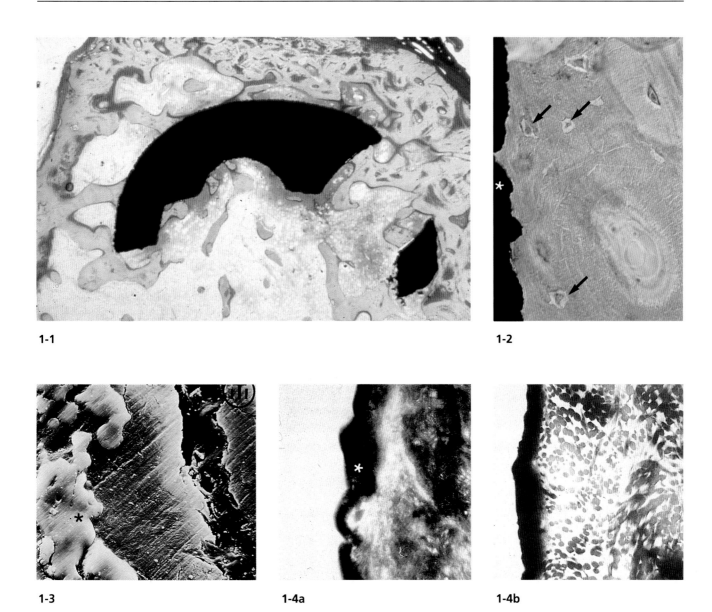

1-1

1-2

1-3

1-4a

1-4b

Fig 1-1   First published scientific evidence of an osseointegrated implant utilizing undecalcified histologic sections. The section demonstrates the direct bone apposition to the prototype hollow-cylinder implant made of titanium. (Reprinted with permission from Schroeder et al.[2])

Fig 1-2   Phenomenon of osseointegration in light microscopic analysis. Direct apposition of bone to a nonsubmerged titanium implant with a rough surface *(asterisk)*. Note the numerous osteocytes *(arrows)* close to the implant surface (beagle dog, 3 months of healing, no functional load).

Fig 1-3   Documentation of osseointegration in SEM analysis. The mineralized bone is in intimate contact with the rough surface of a titanium implant *(asterisk)*.

Figs 1-4a and b   Documentation of osseointegration in TEM analysis utilizing titanium evaporated epoxy implants. Fig 1-4a Direct contact of apatite crystals with the titanium layer *(asterisk)* in an undecalcified section. Fig 1-4b Direct contact of collagen fibrils with the titanium layer *(asterisk)* in a decalcified section. (Original magnifications × 16,000.) Courtesy of M.A. Listgarten, Philadelphia, PA.

Extension of Implant Indications With New Surgical Techniques

One of the most important prerequisites to achieve the above-mentioned success rates with any kind of osseointegrated implants is the presence of a sufficient amount of healthy jawbone at the recipient site. This does not only include an adequate bone height, but also a sufficient crest width.

Clinical studies have clearly demonstrated that the success rate of Brånemark implants is compromised in areas of poor bone quality or in those with good quality but inadequate bone height.[25,26] Screw-type implants with a larger, 5-mm diameter have been recommended for those special situations.[27] An alternative solution for this problem is the use of titanium implants with a rough titanium surface in the bone-anchoring section, such as the TPS surface.[28,29] Experimental studies have indicated that the anchorage of titanium implants with a TPS surface is significantly improved when compared with polished or fine-structured surfaces.[30,31] Thus, titanium implants with a TPS surface, such as ITI implants, have also been successfully utilized in recipient sites with poor bone quality or reduced vertical bone height.[32] In addition, titanium implants with a hydroxyapatite (HA) coating have been recommended for these indications, because the HA coating accelerates bone apposition to the implant surface in the early healing period and significantly improves the anchorage in bone.[33–36] However, several publications have reported that the HA coating is biologically unstable over time and shows signs of resorption in histologic studies.[31,37] This observation might be a contributing factor for the increased rate of complications 3 to 5 years after implant placement, such as severe bone defects around failing or failed HA implants.[38]

New surgical techniques have recently been developed to allow the placement of dental implants in areas with extremely reduced vertical bone height. One of these techniques is the simultaneous use of dental implants with autogenous bone grafts from the iliac crest in severely atrophied mandibles or maxillae.[39–42] In the posterior maxilla, the vertical bone height at potential implant recipient sites is often limited by the extension of the maxillary sinus, and the placement of endosseous implants with a standard technique is not possible. Sinus lift procedures have been recommended to allow the placement of implants even in sites with less than 5 mm of bone height.[43–45] In the posterior mandible, the vertical bone height is limited by the mandibular canal with the neurovascular bundle. To overcome this anatomic limitation, nerve lateralization has been proposed.[46] However, this technique is questionable for routine use in dental offices and appears to be associated with an increased risk for postoperative morbidity, such as dysfunction of the inferior alveolar nerve.[47]

A further problem is the lack of a sufficient crest width. Clinical studies have clearly shown that the long-term prognosis of osseointegrated implants is compromised when the buccal bone wall is missing at the time of implant placement.[48-50] Various surgical techniques have been developed to increase the width of the crest. One of the methods uses a split technique of the narrow alveolar crest and subsequent filling of the created gap between the two cortical bone walls with either autogenous/homologous bone grafts[51,52] or hydroxyapatite.[53,54] The latest surgical technique to improve the volume of jawbone at implant recipient sites involves the principle of guided bone regeneration (GBR). This principle, utilizing barrier membranes, was first evaluated in the late 1950s and early 1960s by the research teams of Bassett et al[55-57] and Boyne et al[58-60] for the healing of cortical defects in long bones and osseous facial reconstruction. These authors utilized microporous cellulose acetate laboratory (Millipore) filters to establish a suitable environment for osteogenesis by excluding connective tissue cells from bone defects. In the early 1980s, this principle was tested in a number of systematic experimental studies for the regeneration of lost periodontal tissues.[61] In implant dentistry, such membranes have been clinically tested in various indications.[62-70] Basics and clinical procedures of this interesting technique are discussed in this book.

Esthetic Considerations

Specific conventional prosthodontic techniques can predictably satisfy esthetic demands of patients with missing teeth (Figs 1-5a and b, 1-6a and b). However, these procedures involve considerably invasive measures, such as the preparation of abutment teeth. Implant-supported restorations, which are less invasive for adjacent teeth, represent a valuable treatment option as long as they provide comparable and long-lasting esthetic results. Because of its obvious biologic advantage, the less invasive approach offered by dental implants is increasingly preferred by many clinicians and patients. To achieve esthetic implant restorations, specific clinical guidelines have been proposed.[71,72] Esthetic implant restorations depend not only on prosthetic and technical aspects, but at least as much on anatomic and surgical aspects.

Anatomic and Surgical Prerequisites for Esthetic Implant Restorations

1. Subgingivally located implant shoulder
2. Adequate implant positioning
3. Stable peri-implant soft tissues
4. Esthetic soft tissue contours

Conventional prosthodontic treatment of congenitally missing anterior teeth. *Figs 1-5 and 1-6*

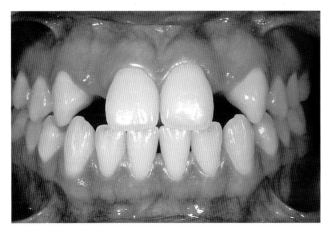

1-5a

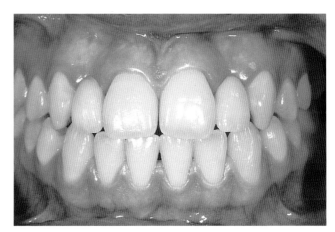

1-5b

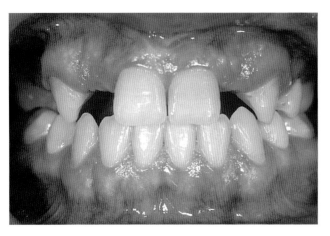

1-6a

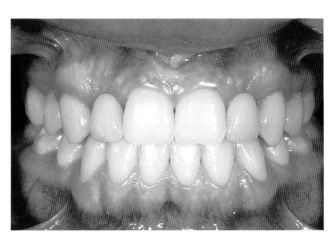

1-6b

Fig 1-5a Young patient with congenitally missing maxillary lateral incisors. Clinical and radiologic examination reveals insufficient vestibular bone volume in the edentulous area and root convergence of the teeth adjacent to the edentulous spaces. Without preoperative measures such as orthodontic therapy and bone augmentation, an implant-supported prosthetic solution is not advisable.

Fig 1-5b Postoperative view after insertion of two three-unit resin-bonded metal-ceramic fixed partial dentures. Maintenance of a harmonious gingival line (regular scalloping) and avoidance of any visible metal are priorities.

Fig 1-6a Preoperative view of a patient with congenitally missing teeth 14, 12, and 22.

Fig 1-6b Final view after cementation of two conventional metal-ceramic fixed partial dentures. The prosthetic restoration includes full coverage for the abutment teeth 16, 13, 23, and 24, as well as two cantilevered units in the region of the maxillary lateral incisors.

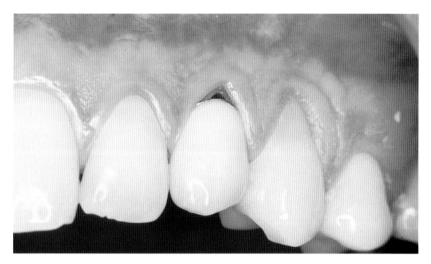

Fig 1-7 Clinical status 5 years after implant placement demonstrating a visible metal margin of an implant-supported single crown.

Within the esthetic zone, a **subgingivally located implant shoulder** is important to avoid any visible cervical metal or margin. In the presence of a high lip line, a visible metal margin (Fig 1-7) is generally considered to be unacceptable. This requires special attention when nonsubmerged ITI implants are utilized. The surgeon must insert the implants deeper into the bone than in standard situations and follow a specific surgical protocol.[73]

Adequate implant positioning is of paramount importance from three points of view. First, the correct implant placement in *orofacial direction* significantly influences the profile of the superstructure. In particular, the point of emergence from the soft tissues determines the final contour of the restoration. A proper emergence profile is generally desirable, both for esthetic and hygienic reasons. Therefore, the projection of the vestibular aspect of the implant shoulder has to emerge as buccally as do adjacent natural teeth. In the presence of localized buccal atrophy, however, implants often have to be placed more palatally in order to insert the implant within the alveolar housing (Figs 1-8a and b). This results in a restoration with a ridge lap design, which can be esthetically pleasing but is clearly more demanding for the patient from a hygienic point of view (Figs 1-8c to f). However, placement of the implant in a more palatal position is limited by the width of the alveolar crest. When the crest width measures less than 5 to 6 mm, a ridge augmentation procedure utilizing the GBR technique is indicated if a dental implant is to be inserted. Second, the correct position of the implant in a *vertical direction* influences (in addition to the above-mentioned esthetically important subgingival location of the implant shoulder) the length of the clinical crown and the accessibility for oral hygiene procedures. In particular, the location of the microgap between the

Restoration with a ridge lap design. *Figs 1-8a to f*

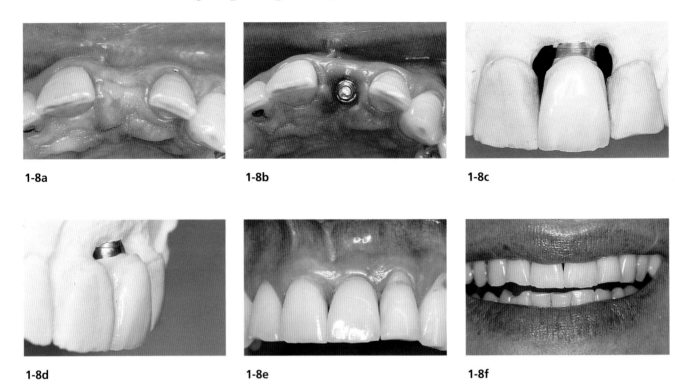

1-8a

1-8b

1-8c

1-8d

1-8e

1-8f

Fig 1-8a Occlusal view of a single-tooth gap in area 21 with buccal atrophy.

Fig 1-8b Buccal atrophy necessitated placement of the ITI implant in a palatal position. Clinical status after completion of the tissue integration period of 3 months.

Fig 1-8c Buccal view of the master cast with the screw-retained single crown mounted onto the implant analog.

Fig 1-8d Lateral view demonstrating the ridge lap design of the single crown to compensate for the palatal position of the implant.

Fig 1-8e Clinical status following insertion of a screw-retained metal-ceramic crown. The ridge lap design allows for an esthetic result.

Fig 1-8f Frontal view of the esthetic result.

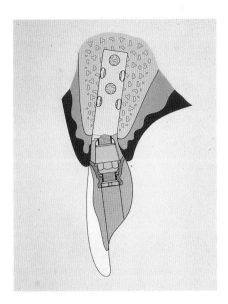

Fig 1-9 Schematic drawing of a 15-degree angled hollow-cylinder implant to compensate for a discrepancy between the implant and the crown axis. (Courtesy of F. Sutter, Waldenburg, Switzerland.)

implant shoulder and the superstructure is of concern from a biologic point of view. In natural dentitions it has been shown that cast restorations with ill-fitting subgingival margins lead to a chronic soft tissue inflammation, probably due in part to a change of the local microbial ecosystem.[74] An implant system providing a precise transfer system and prefabricated copings is therefore favorable in these indications.[75] The third aspect in this context is the *implant axis*, which determines the access to the occlusal screw. Unfortunately, a discrepancy between the potential implant axis and the clinical crown axis is often encountered because of the anatomy of the alveolar process.[71] The screw path might emerge on the facial aspect of the restoration if screw-type implants are placed according to the anatomy of the alveolar ridge. To overcome this, angled abutments have been recommended.[76] A more elegant and less expensive alternative is the use of angled implants, such as the ITI hollow-cylinder implant with a 15-degree angulation (Fig 1-9).[77] In more extreme situations with an extended buccal undercut at potential implant recipient sites, a bone augmentation procedure utilizing the membrane technique is indicated to achieve an appropriate implant axis.

Stable peri-implant soft tissues are essential, since any recession of the mucosa on the buccal aspect of an implant compromises esthetics. Stable soft tissue conditions can be achieved with appropriate home care to maintain a healthy peri-implant mucosa. In addition, the presence of a sufficiently thick (possibly more than 1 mm) buccal bone wall at the time of implant placement is important to support the buccal soft tissues (Fig 1-9). Thus, the width of the alveolar crest is one of the most limiting factors for the placement of an implant. The most prominent implants have diameters between 3 and 4 mm. Therefore, a minimal crest width of 5 to 6 mm has to be present to achieve an intact bone wall of sufficient thickness surrounding the implant. When this minimal crest width is lacking, ridge augmentation is necessary if implants are to be inserted.

Esthetic soft tissue contours, including natural scalloping and distinct papillae, are not only crucial for achieving esthetic results with conventional prostheses,[78] but are also important for implant restorations. In particular, the maintenance of the papillae (Figs 1-10a to d) can be very demanding and requires a proper surgical technique during implant placement.[73]

Summary

Anatomic, surgical, and restorative aspects are important for the achievement of adequate implant restorations that are esthetically acceptable. Careful preoperative site analysis and meticulous surgical techniques, including various methods for site development (GBR, connective tissue grafting, etc), are prerequisites for optimal implant placement and subsequent esthetic restorations. A systematic team approach comprising prosthodontist, implant surgeon, and dental technician is recommended for these demanding implant indications. Utilizing this team approach, esthetically pleasing results can be obtained (Figs 1-11a to d and 1-12a to d).

Restoration of anterior maxillary region with implant-supported crowns. *Figs 1-10 to 1-12*

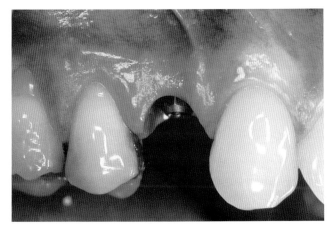

1-10a

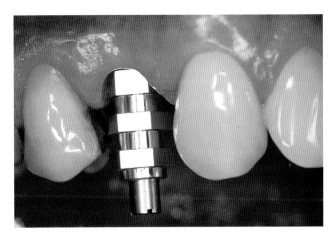

1-10b

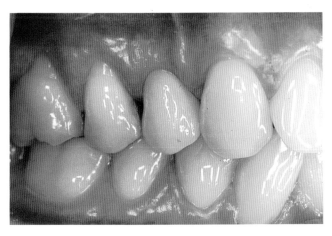

1-10c

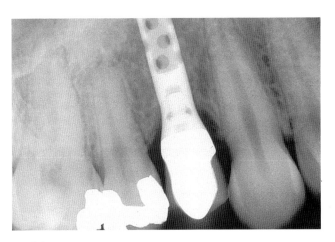

1-10d

Fig 1-10a Clinical status following 3-month tissue-integration period of an ITI implant in area 14. During implant placement, emphasis was given to the maintenance of the papillae.

Fig 1-10b Because of the subgingival implant placement, the ITI implant has to be restored with the Octa System, using precise prefabricated components. The buccal view demonstrates the mounted transfer coping.

Fig 1-10c Buccal view of the implant-supported metal-ceramic crown in area 14. The papillae are maintained, providing an adequate esthetic result.

Fig 1-10d Radiographic follow-up 12 months after implant placement, demonstrating regular peri-implant bone structures.

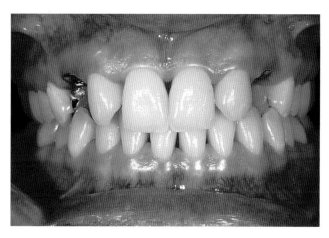

1-11a

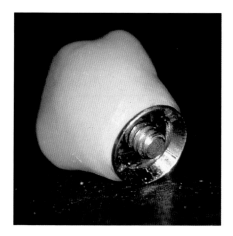

1-11b

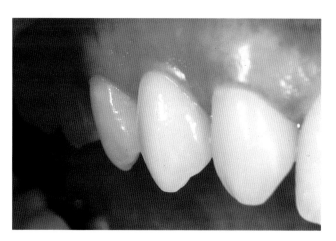

1-11c

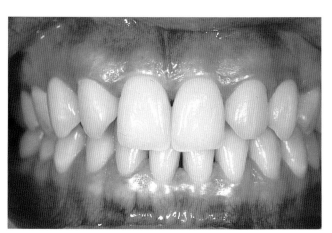

1-11d

Fig 1-11a Patient with bilateral edentulous spaces in the maxillary canine region. Two ITI implants have been inserted.

Fig 1-11b Close-up of a respective screw-retained single-unit restoration using a prefabricated metal coping.

Fig 1-11c Clinical detail of implant site 13. Particular emphasis has been placed on the establishment of a correct emergence profile of the metal ceramic restoration as well as on the maintenance of a harmonious gingival line comprising symmetric papillae.

Fig 1-11d Postoperative frontal view 2 years after placement of implant-supported single-unit restorations in areas 13 and 23.

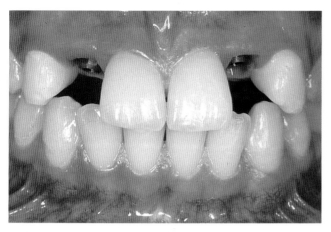

1-12a

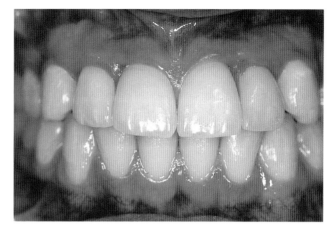

1-12b

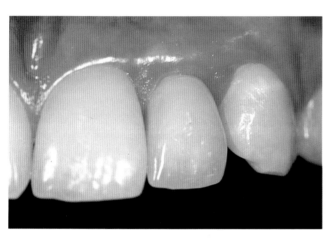

1-12c

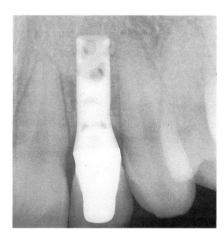

1-12d

Fig 1-12a   Twenty-year-old patient with congenitally missing maxillary lateral incisors. Two ITI implants have been inserted.

Fig 1-12b   Final view after prosthetic rehabilitation. Screw-retained metal-ceramic crowns based on prefabricated copings have been placed in areas 12 and 22.

Fig 1-12c   Detail of the implant-supported metal-ceramic crown in area 22, displaying an adequate emergence profile.

Fig 1-12d   Radiographic follow-up of implant in area 22 two years after implant placement.

Acknowledgment

The professional collaboration of Dr J.-P. Bernard, Dr D. Hess, Dr J.-P. Martinet, Mr B. Eich, Mr M. Magne, and Mr A. Schönenberger during the treatment of the presented cases is highly appreciated.

References

1. Brånemark P-I, Breine U, Adell R, Hansson BO, Lindström J, Olsson A. Intraosseous anchorage of dental prostheses. I. Experimental studies. Scand J Plast Reconstr Surg 1969;3:81.

2. Schroeder A, Pohler O, Sutter F. Gewebsreaktion auf ein Titan-Hohlzylinderimplantat mit Titan-Spritzschichtoberfläche. Schweiz Monatsschr Zahnheilk 1976;86:713.

3. Brånemark P-I, Hansson BO, Adell R, Breine U, Lindström J, Hallen O, Ömann A. Osseo-integrated implants in the treatment of the edentulous jaw. Experience from a 10-year period. Scand J Plast Reconstr Surg 1977;11(suppl 16).

4. Schroeder A, Stich H, Straumann F, Sutter F. Über die Anlagerung von Osteozement an einen belasteten Implantatkörper. Schweiz Monatsschr Zahnheilk 1978;88:1051.

5. Schroeder A, Van der Zypen E, Stich H, Sutter F. The reaction of bone, connective tissue and epithelium to endosteal implants with sprayed titanium surfaces. J Maxillofac Surg 1981;9:15.

6. Listgarten MA, Buser D, Steinemann S, Donath K, Lang NP, Weber HP. Light and transmission electron microscopy of the intact interface between nonsubmerged titanium-coated epoxy resin implants and bone or gingiva. J Dent Res 1992; 71:365.

7. Gotfredsen K, Rostrup E, Hjørting-Hansen E, Stoltze K, Budtz-Jörgensen E. Histological and histomorphometrical evaluation of tissue reactions adjacent to endosteal implants in monkeys. Clin Oral Impl Res 1991;2:30.

8. Weber HP, Buser D, Donath K, Fiorellini JP, Doppolapudi V, Paquette D, Williams RC. Histomorphometry of tissues around submerged and non-submerged implants [abstract]. J Dent Res 1992;71:1198.

9. Brånemark P-I, Zarb GA, Albrektsson T (eds). Tissue-Integrated Prostheses: Osseointegration in Clinical Dentistry. Chicago: Quintessence, 1985.

10. Schroeder A, Sutter F, Krekeler G (eds). Oral Implantology. The ITI Hollow-Cylinder System (English ed). Stuttgart: Georg Thieme Verlag, 1991.

11. Schroeder A, Sutter F, Buser D, Krekeler G (eds). Orale Implantologie. Das ITI System, ed 2. Stuttgart: Georg Thieme Verlag, 1994.

12. Adell R, Lekholm U, Rockler B, Brånemark P-I. A 15-year study of osseointegrated implants in the treatment of the edentulous jaw. Int J Oral Maxillofax Surg 1981;6:387.

13. Adell R, Eriksson B, Lekholm U, Brånemark P-I, Jemt T. A long-term follow-up study of osseointegrated implants in the treatment of totally edentulous jaws. Int J Oral Maxillofac Implants 1990;5:347.

14. Cox JF, Zarb GA. The longitudinal clinical efficacy of osseointegrated dental implants: A 3-year report. Int J Oral Maxillofac Implants 1987;2:91.

15. Zarb GA, Schmitt A. The longitudinal clinical effectiveness of osseointegrated implants. The Toronto study. Part I: Surgical results. J Prosthet Dent 1990;63:451.

16. Babbush CA, Kent JN, Misiek DJ. Titanium plasma-sprayed (TPS) screw implants for the reconstruction of the edentulous mandible. J Oral Maxillofac Surg 1986;44:274.

17. ten Bruggenkate CM, Muller K, Oosterbeek HS. Clinical evaluation of the ITI (F-type) hollow cylinder implant. Oral Surg Oral Med Oral Pathol 1990;70:693.

18. Krekeler G, Schilli W, Geiger H. Das TPS-Implantat, ein zuverlässiges Retentionselement. Z Zahnärztl Implantol 1990;6:229.

19. Buser D, Weber HP, Lang NP. Tissue integration of non-submerged implants. 1-year results of a prospective study with 100 ITI hollow-screw and hollow-cylinder implants. Clin Oral Impl Res 1990;1:33.

20. Buser D, Weber HP, Brägger U, Balsiger C. Tissue integration of one-stage ITI implants: 3-year results of a longitudinal study with hollow-cylinder and hollow-screw implants. Int J Oral Maxillofac Implants 1991;6:405.

21. Buser D, Sutter F, Weber HP, Belser U, Schroeder A. The ITI dental implant system. Basics, clinical indications and procedures, results. In: Hardin J (ed). Clark's Clinical Dentistry, vol 5. Philadelphia: Lippincott, 1992:1–23.

22. Zarb GA, Schmitt A. The longitudinal clinical effectiveness of osseointegrated dental implants in anterior partially edentulous patients. Int J Prosthodont 1993;6:180.

23. Zarb GA, Schmitt A. The longitudinal clinical effectiveness of osseointegrated dental implants in posterior partially edentulous patients. Int J Prosthodont 1993;6:189.

24. Babbush CA, Shimura M. Five-year statistical and clinical observations with the IMZ two-stage osseointegrated implant system. Int J Oral Maxillofac Implants 1993;8:245.

25. Engquist B, Bergendal T, Kallus T, Linden U. A retrospective multicenter evaluation of osseointegrated implants supporting overdentures. Int J Oral Maxillofac Implants 1988;3:129.

26. Jaffin RA, Berman CL. The excessive loss of Brånemark fixtures in type IV bone: A 5-year analysis. J Periodontol 1991;62:2.

27. Langer B, Langer L, Herrmann I, Jorneus L. The wide fixture: A solution for special bone situations and a rescue for the compromised implant. Part 1. Int J Oral Maxillofac Implants 1993;8:400.

28. Hahn H, Palich W. Preliminary evaluation of porous metal surfaced titanium for orthopedic implants. J Biomed Mater Res 1970;4:571.

29. Steinemann S. Titanium. In: Schroeder A, Sutter F, Krekeler G (eds). Oral Implantology. The ITI Hollow-Cylinder System (English ed). Stuttgart: Georg Thieme Verlag, 1991.

30. Wilke HJ, Claes L, Steinemann S. The influence of various titanium surfaces on the interface shear strength between implants and bone. In: Heimke G, Soltész U, Lee AJC (eds). Advances in Biomaterials. Vol 9: Clinical Implant Materials. Amsterdam: Elsevier, 1990:309–314.

31. Buser D, Schenk RK, Steinemann S, Fiorellini J, Fox C, Stich H. Influence of surface characteristics on bone integration of titanium implants. A histomorphometric study in miniature pigs. J Biomed Mater Res 1991;25:889.

32. ten Bruggenkate C. Langzeitergebnisse mit ITI-Implantaten. In: Schroeder A, Sutter F, Buser D, Krekeler G (eds). Orale Implantologie. Das ITI-System, ed 2. Stuttgart: Georg Thieme Verlag, 1994.

33. de Groot K, Geesink R, Klein CPAT, Serekian P. Plasma sprayed coatings of hydroxylapatite. J Biomed Mater Res 1987;21:1375.

34. Thomas KA, Kay JF, Cook SD, Jarcho M. The effect of surface macrotexture and hydroxylapatite coating on the mechanical strengths and histologic profiles of titanium implant materials. J Biomed Mater Res 1987;21:1395.

35. Block MS, Kent JN, Kay JF. Evaluation of hydroxylapatite-coated titanium dental implants in dogs. J Oral Maxillofac Surg 1987;45:601.

36. Block MS, Finger IM, Fontenot MG, Kent JN. Loaded hydroxylapatite-coated and grit-blasted titanium implants in dogs. Int J Oral Maxillofac Implants 1989;4:219.

37. de Lange GL, Donath K. Interface between bone tissue and implants of solid hydroxyapatite or hydroxyapatite-coated titanium implants. Biomaterials 1989;10:121.

38. Johnson BW. HA-coated dental implants: Long-term consequences. CDA J 1992;20:33.

39. Lindström J, Brånemark P-I, Albrektsson T. Mandibular reconstruction using the preformed autologous bone graft. J Plast Reconstr Surg 1981;15:29.

40. Keller EE, Van Roekel NB, Desjardins RP, Tolman DE. Prosthetic-surgical reconstruction of the severely resorbed maxillae with iliac bone grafting and tissue-integrated prostheses. Int J Oral Maxillofac Implants 1987;2:155.

41. Jensen J, Sindet-Pedersen S. Autogenous mandibular bone grafts and osseointegrated implants for reconstruction of the severely atrophic maxilla: A preliminary report. J Oral Maxillofac Surg 1991;49:1277.

42. Weingart D, Strub JR, Schilli W. Mandibular ridge augmentation with autogenous bone grafts and immediate implants. A 3-year longitudinal study. In: Lill W, Spiekermann H, Watzek G (eds). Proceedings of the 5th International Congress on Preprosthetic Surgery. Berlin: Quintessenz, 1993:105.

43. Boyne PJ, James RA. Grafting of the maxillary sinus floor with autogenous marrow and bone. J Oral Surg 1980;38:613.

44. Wood RM, Moore DL. Grafting of the maxillary sinus with intraorally harvested autogenous bone prior to implant placement. Int J Oral Maxillofac Implants 1988;3:209.

45. Kent JN, Block MS. Simultaneous maxillary sinus floor bone grafting and placement of hydroxylapatite coated implants. J Oral Maxillofac Surg 1989;47:238.

46. Jensen OT, Nock D. Inferior alveolar nerve repositioning in conjunction with placement of osseointegrated implants: A case report. Oral Surg Oral Med Oral Pathol 1987;63:263.

47. Friberg B, Ivanoff CJ, Lekholm U. Inferior alveolar nerve transposition in combination with Brånemark implant treatment. Int J Periodont Rest Dent 1992;12:441.

48. Lekholm U, Adell R, Lindhe J, et al. Marginal tissue reactions at osseointegrated titanium fixtures. II: A cross-sectional retrospective study. Int J Oral Maxillofac Surg 1986;15:53.

49. d'Hoedt B. 10 Jahre Tübinger Implantat aus Frialit — Eine Zwischenauswertung der Implantatdatei. Z Zahnärztl Implantol 1986;2:6.

50. Dietrich U, Lippold R, Dirmeier T, Behneke N, Wagner W. Statistische Ergebnisse zur Implantatprognose am Beispiel von 2017 IMZ-Implantaten unterschiedlicher Indikation der letzten 13 Jahre. Z Zahnärztl Implantol 1993;9:9.

51. Streckbein RG, Wöltge E. Augmentationsplastik mit tiefgefrorener homologer Spongiosa als präimplantologische Massnahme beim Einzelzahnersatz. Z Zahnärztl Implantol 1987;3:83.

52. Khoury F. Die modifizierte Alveolar-Extensionsplastik. Z Zahnärztl Implantol 1987;3:174.

53. Osborn JF. Die Alveolar-Extensionsplastik. Quintessenz 1985;36:6701.

54. Nentwig GH, Kniha H. Die Rekonstruktion lokaler Alveolarfortsatzrezessionen im Frontzahnbereich mit Kalziumphosphatkeramik. Z Zahnärztl Implantol 1986;2:80.

55. Hurley LA, Stinchfield FE, Bassett ACL, Lyon WH. The role of soft tissues in osteogenesis. J Bone Joint Surg 1959;41a:1243.

56. Bassett CAL, Creighton DK, Stinchfield FE. Contributions of endosteum, cortex and soft tissues to osteogenesis. Surg Gynecol Obstet 1961;112:145.

57. Bassett CAL. Environmental and cellular factors regulating osteogenesis. In: Frost H (ed). Bone Biodynamics. Boston: Little Brown, 1966:233–244.

58. Boyne PJ. Regeneration of alveolar bone beneath cellulose acetate filter implants. J Dent Res 1964;43:827.

59. Boyne PJ, Mikels TE. Restoration of alveolar ridges by intramandibular transposition osseous grafting. J Oral Surg 1968;26:569.

60. Boyne PJ. Restoration of osseous defects in maxillofacial casualties. J Am Dent Assoc 1969;78:767.

61. Nyman S, Lindhe J, Karring T. Reattachment—new attachment. In: Lindhe J (ed). Textbook of Clinical Periodontology, ed 2. Copenhagen: Munksgard, 1989:450–476.

62. Lazzara RJ. Immediate implant placement into extraction sites: Surgical and restorative advantages. Int J Periodont Rest Dent 1989;9:333.

63. Nyman S, Lang NP, Buser D, Brägger U. Bone regeneration adjacent to titanium dental implants using guided tissue regeneration: A report of two cases. Int J Oral Maxillofac Implants 1990;5:9.

64. Becker W, Becker B. Guided tissue regeneration for implants placed into extraction sockets and for implant dehiscences: Surgical techniques and case reports. Int J Periodont Rest Dent 1990;10:377.

65. Buser D, Brägger U, Lang NP, Nyman S. Regeneration and enlargement of jaw bone using guided tissue regeneration. Clin Oral Impl Res 1990;1:22.

66. Jovanovic S, Spiekermann H, Richter EJ. Bone regeneration around titanium dental implants in dehisced defect sites: A clinical study. Int J Oral Maxillofac Implants 1992;7:233.

67. Buser D, Hirt HP, Dula K, Berthold H. Membrantechnik/Orale Implantologie. Gleichzeitige Anwendung von Membranen bei Implantaten mit periimplantären Knochendefekten. Schweiz Monatsschr Zahnmed 1992;102:1491.

68. Shanaman RH. The use of guided tissue regeneration to facilitate ideal prosthetic placement of implants. Int J Periodont Rest Dent 1992;12:257.

69. Nevins M, Mellonig J. Enhancement of the damaged edentulous ridge to receive dental implants: A combination of allograft and the Gore-Tex membrane. Int J Periodont Rest Dent 1992;12:97.

70. Buser D, Dula K, Belser U, Hirt HP, Berthold H. Localized ridge augmentation using guided bone regeneration. I: Surgical procedure in the maxilla. Int J Periodont Rest Dent 1993;13:29.

71. Parel SM, Sullivan DY. Esthetics and Osseointegration. Dallas: Osseointegration Seminars Inc, Taylor Publishing, 1989.

72. Bahat O. Surgical planning for optimal esthetics and functional results of osseointegrated implants in the partially edentulous mouth. J Calif Dent Assoc 1992;20(5):31.

73. Buser D, Maeglin B. Chirurgisches Vorgehen mit ITI-Implantaten. In: Schroeder A, Sutter F, Buser D, Krekeler G (eds). Orale Implantologie. Das ITI-System, ed 2. Stuttgart: Georg Thieme Verlag, 1994.

74. Lang NP, Kiel RA, Anderhalden K. Clinical and microbiological effects of subgingival restorations with overhanging or clinically perfect margins. J Clin Periodontol 1986;10:563.

75. Sutter F, Weber HP, Sorensen J, Belser U. The new restorative concept of the ITI dental implant system: Design and engineering. Int J Periodont Rest Dent 1993;13:409.

76. Gelb DA, Lazzara R. Hierarchy of objectives in implant placement to maximize esthetics: Use of pre-angulated abutments. Int J Periodont Rest Dent 1993;13:277.

77. Sutter F, Schroeder A, Buser D. The new concept of ITI hollow-cylinder and hollow-screw implants: Part 1. Engineering and design. Int J Oral Maxillofac Implants 1988;3:161.

78. Kopp FR, Belser UC. Esthetic checklist for the fixed prosthesis. In: Schärer P (ed). Esthetic Guidelines for Restorative Dentistry. Chicago: Quintessence, 1982:187–192.

CHAPTER TWO

Scientific Background of Guided Bone Regeneration

Christer Dahlin

The reconstruction of large skeletal deficiencies presents a challenging problem to the orthopedic and surgical community. Such defects in the facial skeleton can be the result of trauma, infection, congenital pseudoarthrosis, or tumor resection. In the reconstructive process, eg, in connection with congenital facial defects, there is often a need to create new bone.

A main hindrance for successful bone healing and for creation of new bone is the rapid formation of soft connective tissue. Ingrowth of soft tissue may disturb or totally prevent osteogenesis in a defect or a wound area. The mechanisms behind the influence of soft connective tissue on osteogenesis are not yet fully understood. Experiments in vitro have demonstrated that fibroblasts produce one or more soluble factors that are inhibitory to bone cell differentiation and osteogenesis.[1] Another possible explanation suggested by Schmitz et al[2] is that a bony non-union development may be due to the failure of the cells that are present to calcify the matrix, perhaps caused by the lack of appropriate bone-derived growth and differentiation factors in large bony defects.

Another frequently occurring clinical situation that causes significant problems for reconstruction is the atrophic edentulous jaw. Since the introduction of reliable oral implant techniques, partially or totally edentulous patients can be successfully treated with jawbone-anchored prostheses.[3,4] However, a prerequisite for the use of oral implants is a sufficient amount of bone to fully cover the implant and to allow the implant to support a fixed prosthetic restoration. Even a minor lack of bone, either horizontal or vertical, may cause a significant problem. A narrow or buccally concave alveolar ridge may result in exposed threads at the alveolar crest or at bone fenestrations. Anatomic restrictions, such as the nasal cavity, maxillary sinuses, and inferior alveolar nerve, in combination with insufficient amounts of bone may dictate a less advantageous placement of the implants, compromising the final restorative result.

Numerous methods have been used in an attempt to solve this problem. One of the most common methods involves the harvesting and implantation of fresh autogenous bone grafts.[5–7] However, this is an expensive procedure that requires hospitalization as well as the potential risk for donor site morbidity. Even though similar methods have been used in more advanced situations of oral reconstructive therapy, only limited scientific data exist regarding the long-term outcome of such treatment.[8] Other methods use bone powder implants or various commercially available allografts.[9,10] Most of these materials act as passive scaffolds, and it is questionable whether such techniques have any real inductive effects on osteogenesis at the cellular level.

In recent years, much research has been focused on the osteogenic potential of demineralized bone powder implants. The stimulatory effects appear to be due to local morphogenic factors inherent in the implanted bone matrix. In general the technique has shown good experimental results,[11,12] but more research is necessary before it can be applied routinely in patients.

Thus, whereas many different methods to improve bone healing and regenerative capacity have been tested, with varying degrees of success, few have reached the stage of routine clinical application. While the future holds promise for new ideas in this area, it is tempered by the realization that the restoration of a deficient skeleton by natural bone remains the ultimate goal.[13]

This chapter reviews the initial animal experiments that have led to the clinical application of guided bone regeneration (GBR) using the membrane technique as a regenerative procedure for bone healing. Different mechanisms, presumably important for the efficacy of membranes to promote osteogenesis, are also discussed.

The Principle of Guided Tissue Regeneration

In the last decade, the principle of guided tissue regeneration (GTR) was developed for regenerating periodontal tissues lost as a result of inflammatory periodontal disease. A series of animal studies, described herein, have documented the possibility of excluding nondesirable cells from populating the wound area by means of membrane barriers and by favoring the proliferation of defined tissue cells to obtain wound healing with a desired type of tissue. New connective tissue fiber attachment and new cementum formation were promoted by excluding dentogingival epithelium and gingival connective tissue proliferation into the wound area adjacent to the root surface, and by creating a space between the inner surface of the membrane and the root surface, giving preference to coronal growth of periodontal ligament cells.

This new approach for reconstructive periodontal therapy has been tested and developed in several clinical studies for a variety of severely compromised periodontal defect types.[14] It has proven to be quite successful for the regeneration of a new attachment apparatus. In many ways it is a scientific and therapeutic breakthrough in periodontal therapy, and logically it has become a widely accepted clinical treatment method.[15]

Development of the Membrane Technique for Bone Regeneration

The principle of physically sealing off an anatomic site for improved healing of a certain tissue type and directing tissue regeneration by some type of mechanical barrier has been used in reconstructive surgery and for neural regeneration since the mid-1950s. For example, microporous cellulose acetate filters were clinically used for nerve and tendon regeneration by Campbell and Bassett[16] as early as 1956 and by Hurley et al[17] in 1959.

The idea of directing host bone into a particular defect is also not a new one. In 1957 Murray et al[18] stated that there were three things necessary for new growth of bone: *(1)* the presence of a blood clot, *(2)* preserved osteoblasts, and *(3)* contact with living tissue. They protected a blood clot with a plastic fenestrated cage, and the interior of the cage became filled with bone. Linghorne[19] showed that it was possible to bridge a 15-mm gap, prepared in the fibula of a dog, using a polyethylene tube filled with a blood clot and autogenous cancellous grafts. A similar control defect demonstrated a fibrous repair.

Melcher and Dreyer[20] also found evidence for the importance of preserving the blood clot. They studied the healing process of a penetrating defect in the rat's femur, where the blood clot was protected with either a plastic or organic shield during healing. The study's conclusion suggested that the role of the shield is twofold: *(1)* it protects the hematoma from invasion by non-osteogenic shields, and *(2)* it governs the size of the

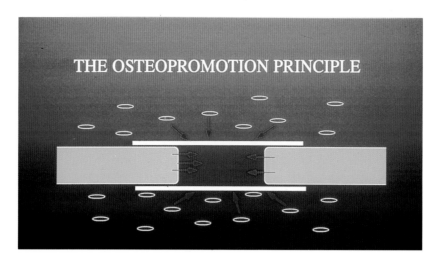

Fig 2-1 Ilustration of the placement of mechanical barriers (membranes) to seal off the bone defect from the surrounding soft connective tissue. This creates a secluded space into which cells only from the surrounding bone can migrate.

hematoma and prevents its distortion by the pressure of the overlying tissue. It has also been shown that the placement of cellulose acetate filters can improve the regeneration of alveolar bone defects in dogs.[21] Furthermore, it has been used clinically, as a lining of implanted metallic cages, filled with autogenous marrow and bone for the restoration of jaw defects.[22]

These concepts were also evaluated experimentally by Kahnberg in 1979.[23] He studied the healing process in mandibular base defects in rabbits with subperiosteally implanted Teflon mantle leafs, and stated that the mantle leafs prevented ingrowth of fibrous scar tissue, allowing bone regeneration to occur.

Experimental studies performed in various animal models have proven that the mechanical barrier principle, although different in many respects, is also applicable in osseous reconstructive surgery. The concept implies that placement of a barrier membrane prevents ingrowth of soft connective tissue into bone defects. The membrane is placed in direct contact with the surrounding bone surface, thereby placing the periosteum on the outer surface of the membrane. The mucoperiosteal flap is then repositioned and sutured, creating a closed situation (Fig 2-1).

Osteopromotion is a term found frequently in the literature to describe the use of physical means to seal off an anatomic site—the site where the bone is intended to be (re)formed—to prevent other tissues, notably soft connective tissue, from interfering with osteogenesis as well as to direct bone formation. This terminology is in accordance with earlier designations used to describe different mechanisms that characterize the osteogenic process, eg, ostenconduction, osteoinduction, and osseointegration.[24]

The best documented membrane material for this purpose is expanded polytetrafluoroethylene (e-PTFE). This material is inert and has an extensive history of use in clinical medicine (see Chapter 4).

The use of e-PTFE material for osteopromotion is well illustrated in a paper published in 1988 by Dahlin et al,[25] who raised mucoperiosteal flaps and produced bilateral bone defects in the mandibles of 30 adult rats. On one side the defect was covered with an e-PTFE membrane (Gore-Tex, W.L. Gore, Flagstaff, AZ), while on the other side the defect was only covered with the muscle-periosteal flap (Figs 2-2a and b). The results, obtained by gross and histomorphometric analysis, showed that the mechanical hindrance of growth of fibrous connective tissue cells into the bone defects resulted in a virtually complete bone healing of the test sites, whereas the control defects were filled with fibrous connective tissue with only minor ingrowth of new bone at the defect margins (Figs 2-2c to f). The profound importance of mechanical hindrance to soft connective tissue proliferation for bone healing was clearly demonstrated.

Furthermore, the chemical and biologic inertness of the e-PTFE membranes used was demonstrated by the lack of adverse tissue reactions. In subsequent experiments,[26] the tissue healing dynamics in the rat mandibular defect were characterized. Incorporation of [3H]-thymidine, a marker for cell division, demonstrated mitotic activity 10 days after surgery in endosseous cells within the bone, adjacent to membrane-covered defects. Incorporation of 45Ca, a chemical assay for bone mineralization, into newly formed bone was significantly lower in control defects, yielding a maximal incorporation after 2 weeks of healing. At sites where membranes had been placed, mineralization was found to get underway somewhat later but showed a steady increase in incorporation during the first weeks, with maximal activity at 5 weeks after surgery (Fig 2-3).

The presence of growth factors related to bone healing could be demonstrated within the healing defects. Finally, the incorporation pattern of fluorochromes corroborated the impression that the placement of membranes slowed the onset of bone regeneration (the beginning of osteogenesis taking place nearly 2 weeks after surgery) but led to a complete bony restitution of the defects. However, the results obtained are not necessarily transferable to the human situation, since the rat is a low phylogenetic species with a high potential for osteogenesis.

For this reason, another study was performed using primates.[27] Bilateral, transosseous defects were created in edentulous areas of the mandible, and in the maxilla in conjunction with an apicoectomy procedure of the lateral incisors. One side served as the test site, with membranes placed buccally and palatally, entirely covering the entrances to the defects. The contralateral sides,

Fig 2-2a   Experimental model of a transosseous defect (5 mm in diameter) surgically created bilaterally through the mandibular angles of a rat.

Fig 2-2b   In the test defects, the buccal and lingual entrances to the transosseous defects are covered by an e-PTFE membrane that is secured in place by a transosseous suture prior to repositioning of the mucoperiosteal flaps. In control defects, the same procedure is followed but without the placement of a membrane.

Fig 2-2c   Gross appearance of the control defect (no membrane) of a representative animal after 9 weeks of healing. The defect is still not ossified, although it is somewhat diminished in diameter.

Fig 2-2d   Test site (membrane-covered) after 9 weeks, demonstrating solid bone healing. Note the increase in cortical bone mass.

Fig 2-2e   Photomicrograph showing bone healing after 6 weeks in one representative animal (test site). The margins of the original defect are indicated with arrows in the histologic section (nb = new bone, m = membrane). Hematoxylin and eosin stain; original magnification × 125.

Fig 2-2f   After 6 weeks of healing without a membrane, the defect is mainly filled with soft connective tissue. Only minor apposition of newly formed bone is seen at the margins of the defect (arrows indicate the original defect margins, ct = connective tissue). Hematoxylin and eosin stain; original magnification × 125.

Use of e-PTFE membrane in an experimental study in adult rats.[25]   *Figs 2-2a to f*

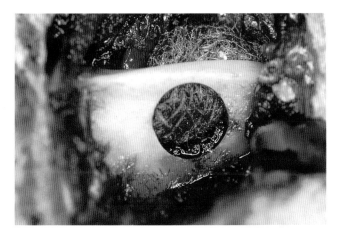

2-2a

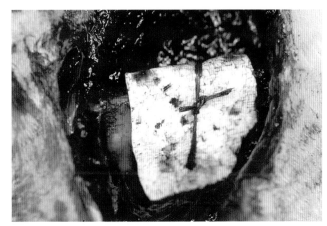

2-2b

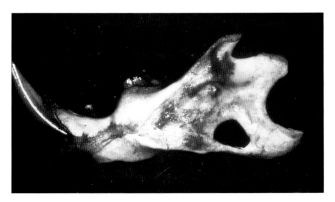

2-2c

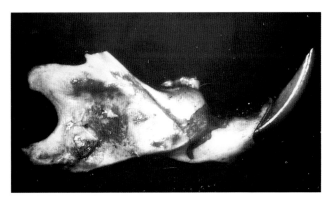

2-2d

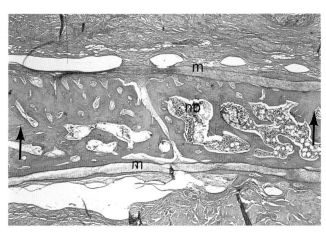

2-2e

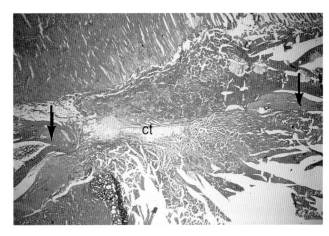

2-2f

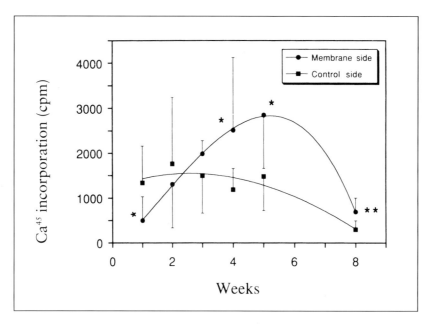

Fig 2-3 Incorporation of 45Ca into the bone mineral phase at the defect sites, demonstrating the rate of mineralization at certain points in time after surgery. The results are expressed as counts per minute (cpm; mean values ± SD) as a function of the healing period (weeks). The rate of isotope incorporation at the membrane-treated sites was significantly lower 1 week after surgery compared to the control defects, whereas it was significantly higher at the 4-, 5- and 8-week examinations.

without the placement of membranes, served as controls (Figs 2-4a to d). A total of 12 animals were included in the study. There was complete regeneration of the transosseous defects treated with membranes in the mandible and the maxilla. The control defects in the mandible and the maxilla showed little or no bone healing; instead, the defects were mainly filled with a trans-osseous connective tissue core with collagen fibers running throughout the defect (Figs 2-4e to h).

The membrane technique has not only been shown to regenerate bone in bony defects. Linde et al[28] demonstrated that the osteopromotive membrane concept had the capability to actually form bone at anatomic sites where there should not be any bone present. They used a stiffer "dome"-shaped membrane material, which was placed on top of the flat calvarium of rats, creating a secluded space into which osteogenic cells from the calvarial bone could migrate. Extra care was taken to secure a blood clot beneath the membrane. Predictable bone neogenesis could be seen in this model.

Recently, Schmid et al[29] reported similar findings, with bone neogenesis on top of a flat bone surface, when testing a novel implant system in combination with e-PTFE membranes.

Membrane study conducted in primates.[27]

Figs 2-4a to h

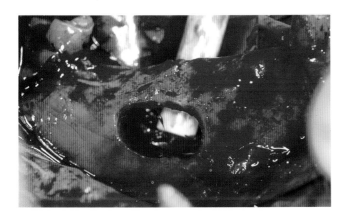

2-4a

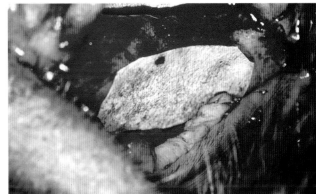

2-4b

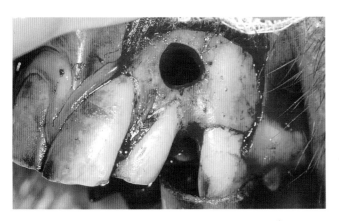

2-4c

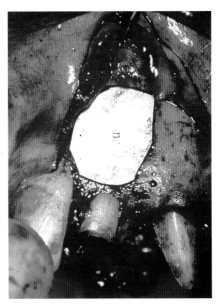

2-4d

Fig 2-4a   Transosseous defect (8 × 12 mm) surgically created bilaterally in the mandible of monkeys.

Fig 2-4b   Placement of buccally and lingually placed e-PTFE membranes as mechanical barriers, totally covering the entrances to the mandibular defect.

Fig 2-4c   Similar procedure was accomplished in the maxilla. Transosseous defects with a diameter of 10 mm were created bilaterally in a buccopalatal direction. The photograph shows a control defect (without the placement of membranes).

Fig 2-4d   Buccally placed membrane (e-PTFE) completely covering the entrance to the defect.

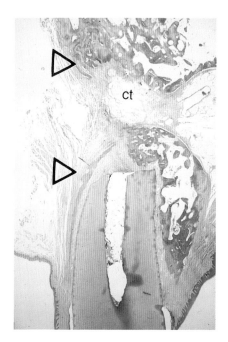

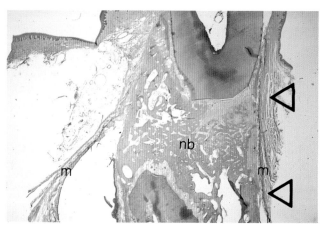

Fig 2-4e Control defect in the maxilla (no membranes) 3 months postoperatively. The defect is virtually filled with dense soft connective tissue. The collagen fibers are running at right angles to the buccal and palatal bone surfaces. (Arrowheads indicate the osseous defect; ct = connective tissue.) Hematoxylin and eosin stain; original magnification × 30.

Fig 2-4f Membrane-covered defect in the maxilla after 3 months of healing. The defect is almost completely filled with newly formed trabecular bone. A minute soft tissue portion of connective tissue is seen at the apex of the apicoectomized tooth. (Arrowheads indicate the buccal entrance to the defect; ct = connective tissue, nb = new bone, m = membrane.) Hematoxylin and eosin stain; original magnification × 80.

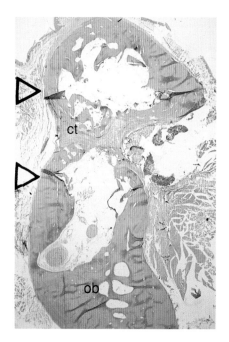

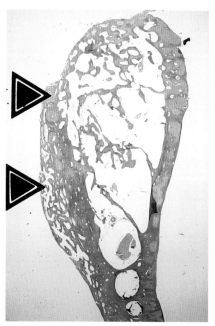

Fig 2-4g Mandibular control defect (no membrane). Note the lack of continuity of the compact bone layer and the presence of the transosseous "core" of dense connective tissue. (Arrowheads indicate the original defect; ct = connective tissue, ob = original bone.) Hematoxylin and eosin stain; original magnification × 30.

Fig 2-4h Complete bone healing on the test (membrane) side in the mandible after a healing period of 3 months. The original margins of the defect are indicated by arrowheads. Note also the apposition of new bone on the outside of the mandible beneath the membrane. Hematoxylin and eosin stain; original magnification × 25.

2-4g

2-4h

How Guided Bone Regeneration Works

Guided bone regeneration has proven to be successful in a variety of experimental animal models. However, little is found in the literature about the underlying basic mechanisms behind the concept. In general, it has been stated that new bone formation develops from the periosteum and marrow-derived cells showing osteogenic potential.

The effect of the placement of mechanical barriers on the early healing phase in a wound situation needs to be better understood. It has been speculated that such a procedure facilitates recruitment of cells with osteogenic potential from cell populations in haversian and Volkmann's canals, and mostly from the endosteum. Thus, the periosteum is excluded because it is readapted on the outer surface of the membranes.

The experimental studies summarized above have proven that certain tissues within the body possess the biologic potential for regeneration if the proper environment is provided during healing. The ultimate goal of guided bone regeneration is to use a temporary device to provide the necessary environment that allows the body to utilize its natural healing potential and regenerate lost and absent tissue.

Even though this explanation certainly is of great importance, the efficacy of membranes in conjunction with bone healing and reconstructive therapy is probably the result of a combination of different mechanisms—mechanical, cellular, and molecular.[24] Examples of these are:

- Prevention of fibroblast mass action
- Prevention of contact inhibition by heterotopic cell interaction
- Exclusion of cell-derived soluble inhibitory factors
- Local concentration of growth stimulatory factors
- Stimulatory properties of the membrane itself

These studies have also shown that the sequence of healing occurring in fracture repair follows the same basic patterns that are found during healing of an osseous lesion during guided bone regeneration therapy (see Chapter 3).

Bone Augmentation Around Dental Implants

Successful rehabilitation of edentulism with the use of oral implants requires complete bone coverage of the implants. This would mean that a minimum of 7 × 4 mm of bone tissue is needed when the smallest type of implant for oral application is used. Finding an alternative to more resource-demanding bone grafting procedures for the treatment of localized bone defects has therefore been of great interest.

Based on the findings of the studies summarized above, Dahlin et al[30] placed endosseous implants bilaterally into the tibiae of rabbits. The implants were placed in such a way that three to four threads were left exposed on one side, simulating an osseous defect adjacent to an implant. Half of the implants placed were covered with an e-PTFE membrane, creating a space between the membrane, the implant, and a portion of the adjacent cortical bone of the tibia. The implant helped provide support for the membrane and could thus create the necessary space for new bone formation to occur. The other half of the implants, inserted in the contralateral tibia, served as controls (Figs 2-5a and b). All membrane-treated sites predictably showed

Fig 2-5a In each animal, two fixtures (one in each tibia) were placed in such a way that three to four of the coronal threads were left exposed on one side of each implant.

Fig 2-5b Covering of the implant with a membrane. In each animal, one fixture (test) was covered with an e-PTFE membrane extending 5 to 8 mm around the fixture. The periosteal flap was adapted on the outer surface of the membrane to allow full coverage and stabilization of the membrane.

Fig 2-5c and d Bone healing adjacent to titanium implants. Longitudinal ground sections (10 μm thick) represent the midportion of the fixtures. The sections were stained with toluidine blue/pyronin G. Histologic measurements were made from the original bone crest after preparation of the implant site (ob) to the reference point on the fixture (rp), as well as from the original bone crest (ob) to the crest of the newly formed bone (nb). The results were expressed as percent gain of bone cover. Fig 2-5c demonstrates bone healing on the control side (no membrane) and Fig 2-5d the test site after 6 weeks of healing. Original magnification × 40.

Fig 2-5e Newly formed bone adjacent to implant after 6 weeks of healing on the test (membrane) side. Deposition of bone (B) into the threads of the implant (im) is evident. Numerous osteoblasts can be seen. Osseointegration is evident, as indicated by light microscopy. Ground section, toluidine blue/pyronin G stain; original magnification × 500.

Membranes used in conjunction with implants in rabbit tibiae.[30] *Figs 2-5a to e*

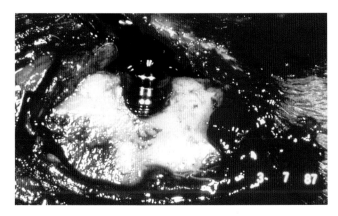

2-5a

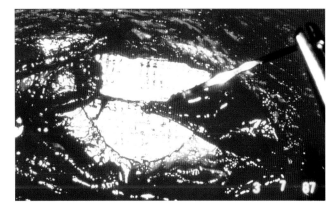

2-5b

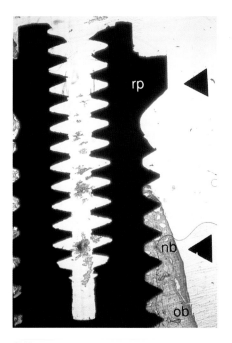

2-5c

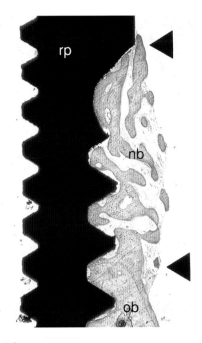

2-5d

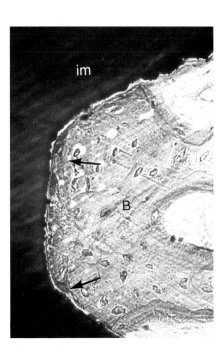

2-5e

new bone formation in the space provided by the membrane (mean 99.5%, range 95.6% to 100%). This bone growth was significantly (P < .0001) greater than that measured at the control sites (mean 66.4%, range 38.9% to 92.4%) using photometric measurements. The majority of the new bone was created within 6 weeks (Figs 2-5c and d). In addition, a direct contact between the newly formed bone and the titanium surface of the implants was observed (Fig 2-5e). The authors concluded that a complete selective formation of bone within a defined bone defect can be accomplished by preventing cells not derived from the surrounding bone from populating the defect area.

Those initial findings were further supported by several experimental studies. Becker et al[31] tested the membrane technique in conjunction with endosseous implants at mandibular sites in dogs. Implants were placed in such a way that the fixture head and the adjacent threads remained above the horizontal bone level. Half of the implants placed were covered with e-PTFE membranes. A few complications, such as soft tissue perforations, occurred—most likely a result of fixture positioning. Thus, within the limitations of the study afforded by these complications, the data clearly revealed the potential of the membrane technique for forming new bone around dental implants.

Using experimentally produced dehiscence defects (3 × 5 mm) in canine models, Zablotsky et al[32] showed enhanced bone regeneration (mean 95.17% over HA-coated implants, 82.8% over grit-blasted titanium implants) compared to nonmembrane controls when using e-PTFE membranes in conjunction with endosseous implants. An additional important finding of this study was that guided bone regeneration seems to function as a general principle regardless of the implant system used.

Immediate placement of implants into fresh extraction sockets combined with the use of membranes is another area that may offer a number of advantages from a clinical standpoint (see Chapter 5). This procedure may protect the ridge from resorbing. If ridge height and width can be preserved, longer implants can be placed, thereby increasing the supporting bone volume contacting the implant. Furthermore, immediate implant placement into extraction sites may shorten the time necessary to complete the restorative phase of treatment. Becker et al[33] conducted a study in dogs in simulated extraction sites. Six Brånemark implants were protected by e-PTFE membranes and six additional implants served as controls without membrane application. Clinical and histologic evaluations were performed after 18 weeks of healing. The membrane-covered implants demonstrated an average bone gain of 2.6 mm, while the controls revealed an average of 1.0 mm. The authors concluded that, "Implants augmented with e-PTFE membranes had clinically significant higher amounts of bone regeneration when compared with [nonmembrane] controls."

Warrer et al[34] used e-PTFE membranes to treat extraction socket defects adjacent to endosseous implants in seven monkeys. The maxillary second molars were selected as experimental sites and were extracted as atraumatically as possible. The largest of the three root sockets was selected for insertion of 8-mm screw-type implants. Prior to suturing, an occlusive membrane was adjusted to cover half of the implants placed and their surrounding bony craters. Light microscopic analysis after 3 months of healing revealed a varying degree of soft tissue facing the coronal portion of the control (nonmembrane) implants, whereas osseointegration was consistently seen to the top of the membrane-covered implants.

A technical problem encountered when bony defects around dental implants are treated with the GBR technique is that several types of defects are not naturally spacemaking. This is often the case when implants are placed into areas with inadequate bone volume (ie, dehiscence defects in conjunction with the fixture head, certain fenestration defects, or residual intraosseous defects) or into extraction sockets. Several space-maintaining materials have been proposed for use in conjunction with the membrane technique. However, from a biologic point of view, the best material is fresh autogenous bone, harvested from the actual surgical site of the patient. This suggestion has been confirmed in a study by Dahlin et al,[35] who reported successful bone healing of 8-mm cranial defects in adult rats by the use of membranes and interpositioned autogenous bone chips. Furthermore, no osteoinductive potential from the bone chips was observed. They were mainly serving as "tent poles" between the membranes.

In conjunction with the placement of screw-type implants, Gotfredsen et al[36] used porous hydroxyapatite (HA, Interpore 200 granules, Interpore International) with or without membranes (Gore-Tex Augmentation Material, W.L. Gore) in bony defects of monkeys. The study comprised four test groups: *(1)* membrane only, *(2)* grafting with HA and membrane, *(3)* grafting with HA only, and *(4)* no treatment (control).

After 12 weeks of healing, all peri-implant bone defects treated with membranes and those with a combination of HA and membranes were completely filled with new bone. The defects treated with HA alone and the control defects with no treatment demonstrated only new bone formation at the bottom of the defects. The authors concluded that the membrane technique provides possibilities for healing of bone defects around endosseous dental implants. The HA alone did not promote bone regeneration and had no additional effect on bone healing when combined with the GBR technique.

Another experimental study using synthetic graft material that is of potential clinical interest was performed by Seibert and Nyman.[37] They combined the membrane technique and porous HA blocks (Interpore 200) in an attempt to perform a ridge augmentation procedure in edentulous maxillae in dogs. Complete bone fill in those sites where membranes had been combined with the HA strut was found after 90 days of healing. The sham-operated (control) sites did not undergo repair and bone fill even after an observation period of 180 days.

Summary

This chapter has provided an overview of the experimental studies that have served as a basis for the introduction of guided bone regeneration into clinical practice. Based on these studies and on sound scientific evidence, it can be stated that certain conditions must be met for new bone formation to be predictably accomplished by guided bone regeneration:

1. There must be a source of osteogenic cells. Viable bone must be present adjacent to the defect where regeneration is desired.
2. An adequate source of vascularity is essential. This supply comes mostly from the adjacent bone surface (Volkmann's canals and marrow compartments).
3. The wound site must remain mechanically stable during healing.
4. An appropriate space must be created and maintained between the membrane and the parent bone surface.
5. Soft connective tissue cells must be excluded from the space created by the membrane barrier. The structure of the material used must be able to accomplish this.

It must be emphasized that no one knows for certain whether e-PTFE is a membrane material with unique characteristics. Today it is by far the best experimentally evaluated material used exclusively for bone regenerative purposes. When introducing the concept of guided bone regeneration into clinical practice, the five conditions mentioned above must be met. In addition, the fundamental biologic principles of bone healing, appropriate surgical techniques, an appropriately designed membrane material, and, last but not least, careful patient selection need to be taken into account.

References

1. Ogiso B, Hughes FJ, Melcher AC, McCulloch CAG. Fibroblasts inhibit mineralized bone nodule formation by rat bone marrow stromal cells in vitro. J Cell Physiol 1991;146:442.

2. Schmitz JP, Schwartz Z, Hollinger JO, Boyan B. Characterization of rat calvarial nonunion defects. Acta Anat 1990;138:185.

3. Adell R, Lekholm U, Brånemark P-I. Surgical procedures. In: Brånemark P-I, Zarb GA, Albrektsson T (eds). Tissue-Integrated Prostheses: Osseointegration in Clinical Dentistry. Chicago: Quintessence, 1985:211–232.

4. Adell R, Eriksson B, Lekholm U, Brånemark P-I, Jemt T. A long-term follow-up study of osseointregrated implants in the treatment of the totally edentulous jaw. Int J Oral Maxillofac Implants 1990;4:347.

5. Keller EE, Van Roekel NB, Desjardins RP, Tolman DE. Prosthetic-surgical reconstruction of the severely resorbed maxilla with iliac bone grafting. Int J Oral Maxillofac Implants 1987;2:155.

6. Kahnberg K-E, Nyström E, Bartholdsson L. Combined use of bone grafts and Brånemark fixtures in the treatment of severely resorbed maxillae. Int J Oral Maxillofac Implants 1989;4:297.

7. Adell R, Lekholm U, Gröndahl K, Brånemark P-I, Lindström J, Jacobsson M. Reconstruction of severely resorbed edentulous maxillae using osseointegrated fixtures in immediate autogenous bone grafts. Int J Oral Maxillofac Implants 1990;5:233.

8. Oklund S, Prolo DJ, Gutierrez RV, et al. Quantitative comparisons of healing in cranial fresh autografts, frozen autografts and processed autografts, and allografts in canine skull defects. Clin Orthop 1986;205:269.

9. Jarcho M. Retrospective analysis of hydroxyapatite development for implant applications. Dent Clin North Am 1992; 36:19.

10. Kent JN, Zide MF. Bone and biomaterials. Otolaryngol Clin North Am 1984;17:273.

11. Kaban LB, Glowacki J. Induced osteogenesis in the repair of mandibular defects in rats. J Dent Res 1981;60:1356.

12. Glowacki J, Kaban LB, Murray JE, Folkman J, Mulliken JB. Application of the biological principle of induced osteogenesis for craniofacial defects. Lancet 1981;2:959.

13. Prolo DJ, Rodrigo JJ. Contemporary bone graft physiology and surgery. Clin Orthop 1985;200:322.

14. Nyman S, Lindhe J, Karring T. Reattachment—New Attachment. In: Lindhe J (ed). Textbook of Clinical Periodontology. Copenhagen: Munskgaard, 1988:409–429.

15. Gottlow J, Nyman S, Karring T. Maintenance of new attachment gained through guided tissue regeneration. J Clin Periodontol 1992;19:315.

16. Campbell JB, Bassett CAL. The surgical application of monomolecular filters (Millipore) to bridge gaps in peripheral nerves and to prevent neuroma formation. Surg Forum 1956;7:570.

17. Hurley AL, Stinchfield FE, Bassett CAL, Lyon WH. The role of soft tissues in osteogenesis. J Bone Joint Surg 1959;41A:1243.

18. Murray G, Holden R, Roachlau W. Experimental and clinical study of new growth of bone in a cavity. Am J Surg 1957;93:385.

19. Linghorne WJ. The sequence of events in osteogenesis as studied in polyethylene tubes. Ann NY Acad Sci 1960;xy:445.

20. Melcher AH, Dreyer CJ. Protection of the blood clot in healing circumscribed bone defects. J Bone Joint Surg 1962;44B:424.

21. Boyne PJ. Regeneration of alveolar bone beneath cellulose acetate filter implants [abstract]. J Dent Res 1964;43:827.

22. Boyne PJ. Restoration of osseous defects in maxillofacial casualties. J Am Dent Assoc 1969;78:767.

23. Kahnberg K-E. Restoration of mandibular jaw defects in the rabbit by sub-periosteally implanted Teflon mantle leaf. Int J Oral Surg 1979;8:449.

24. Linde A, Alberius P, Dahlin C, Bjurstam K, Sundin Y. Osteopromotion: A soft-tissue exclusion principle using a membrane for bone healing and bone neogenesis. J Periodontol (in press).

25. Dahlin C, Linde A, Gottlow J, Nyman S. Healing of bone defects by guided tissue regeneration. Plast Reconstr Surg 1988;81:672.

26. Dahlin C. Osteopromotion: Regeneration of Bone by a Membrane Technique [thesis]. Gothenburg, Sweden, 1993.

27. Dahlin C, Gottlow J, Linde A, Nyman S. Healing of maxillary and mandibular bone defects using a membrane technique. An experimental study in monkeys. Scand J Plast Reconstr Surg Hand Surg 1990;24:13.

28. Linde A, Thorén C, Dahlin C, Sanberg E. Creation of new bone by an osteopromotive membrane technique. An experimental study in rats. J Oral Maxillofac Surg (in press).

29. Schmid J, Hämmerle CHF, Stich H, Lang NP. Supraplant®, a novel implant system based on the principle of guided bone regeneration. Clin Oral Impl Res 1991;2:199.

30. Dahlin C, Sennerby L, Lekholm U, Linde A, Nyman S. Generation of new bone around titanium implants using a membrane technique: An experimental study in rabbits. Int J Oral Maxillofac Implants 1989;4:19.

31. Becker W, Becker BE, Handlesman M, Celletti R, Ochsenbein C, Hardwick R, Langer B. Bone formation at dehisced dental implant sites treated with implant augmentation material: A pilot study in dogs. Int J Periodont Rest Dent 1990;10:93.

32. Zablotsky M, Meffert R, Caudill R, Evans G. Histological and clinical comparisons of guided tissue regeneration on dehisced hydroxyapatite-coated and titanium endosseous implant surfaces. Int J Oral Maxillofac Implants 1991;6:294.

33. Becker W, Becker B, Handelsman M, Ochsenbein C, Albrektsson T. Guided tissue regeneration for implants placed into extraction sockets. A study in dogs. J Periodontol 1991;62:703.

34. Warrer K, Gotfredsen K, Hjørting-Hansen E, Karring T. Guided tissue regeneration ensures osseointegration of dental implants placed into extraction sockets. An experimental study in monkeys. Clin Oral Impl Res 1991;2:166.

35. Dahlin C, Alberius P, Linde A. Osteopromotion for cranioplasty. An experimental study in rats using a membrane technique. J Neurosurg 1991;74:487.

36. Gotfredsen K, Warrer K, Hjørting-Hansen E, Karring T. Effect on membranes and HA on healing in osseous craters around titanium implants. Clin Oral Impl Res 1991;2:172.

37. Seibert J, Nyman S. Localized ridge augmentation in dogs. A pilot study using membranes and hydroxyapatite. J Periodontol 1990;61:157.

CHAPTER THREE

Bone Regeneration: Biologic Basis

Robert K. Schenk

Bone is considered to be the highest achievement in the evolution of supporting tissues. A first and decisive step in this evolution was the elaboration of collagen fibers in the connective tissues. They offer superb tensile strength but cannot resist other sorts of deformation and, therefore, cannot maintain a given shape. Cartilage solved this problem by extruding proteoglycans into the interfibrillar space. Trapped within the collagen network, the osmotic or electrostatic swelling capacity of proteoglycans provides an extracellular matrix with the elasticity to withstand compression and shear forces. The final step toward a solid building material, however, was mineralization. Calcified cartilage was the first attempt in this direction. Calcium phosphate and hydroxyapatite are precipitated in the interfibrillar space formerly occupied by proteoglycans. This mineralized filler stiffens the cartilaginous matrix but also impedes the transport of nutrients to the entrapped cells. This was a severe handicap for the construction of large skeletal components. In bone, the formation of intercellular connections via cytoplasmic processes allowed transport of metabolites from the lining cells on the surface to the deeper osteocytes and a further increase in mineral density. Finally, the direct association between apatite crystals and collagen fibrils further improved mechanical properties.

Besides its excellent mechanical behavior, bone reveals a unique potential for regeneration. Bone is able to heal fractures or local defects with regenerated tissue, or "regenerate," of equally high structural organization, without leaving a scar.

The mechanism of this healing pattern is often considered as a recapitulation of embryonic osteogenesis and growth. The aim of this chapter, therefore, is to summarize the basic facts of development, structure, and function of bone in order to provide the biologic basis for discussion of the pattern of guided bone regeneration.

Bone Structure

Macroscopic Structure

Long bones are subdivided into epiphysis, metaphysis, and diaphysis regions. Epiphyses and metaphyses are characterized by a compact cortical layer that surrounds a body of spongy bone consisting of trabeculae, either in the shape of rods or plates. Toward the diaphysis, the cortical bone becomes thicker and the trabeculae are replaced by a coherent marrow cavity.

In small bones, such as vertebrae, carpal, and tarsal bones, there is no diaphysis and the metaphyses have merged. Ribs, the mandible, and certain parts of the skull also consist of cancellous bone surrounded by a cortical layer.

The mineralized structure of bone is enclosed by the periosteal and endosteal **envelopes**. The vascular canals within compact bone are continuations of the periosteal or endosteal envelopes (endocortical or haversian envelope). All three envelopes share two important features: osteogenic potential and abundant vascularization. This enables the envelopes to participate in modeling and remodeling activities, as well as in bone repair. The periosteum covers the outer surface of the bones, with the exception of the articular surfaces and tendon and ligament insertions. Its structure varies from delicate, loose connective tissue sheets to dense fibrous membranes. Osteoprogenitor cells are commonly located in the vicinity of blood vessels near the bone surface. The cells of the endosteum belong to the stroma of the bone marrow or are derived from resting osteoblasts, which also constitute the main source of lining cells in the cortical canals.

Microscopic Structure

Based on the orientation of the collagen fibrils, three types of bone tissue are distinguished: woven bone, lamellar bone, and an intermediate type—the primary parallel-fibered bone.[1] The texture of the collagen fibrils was originally analyzed in polarized light and later visualized by electron microscopy.

In **woven bone**, the collagen fibrils are oriented in a random or feltlike manner. Woven bone is formed predominantly in embryos and growing children, and is later replaced by lamellar bone. In the adult, it reappears when accelerated bone formation is required, as in the bony callus during fracture repair and in pathologic conditions like Paget's disease, renal osteodystrophy, hyperparathyroidism, or fluorosis. Besides its interlacing fibrils, woven bone is characterized by more numerous and larger osteocytes and, in microradiographs, by its high mineral density. Fluorochrome labeling results in a diffuse rather than in a clearly delineated uptake.

Lamellar bone is characterized by 3- to 5-μm-wide layers of parallel collagen fibrils. The orientation of the fibrils changes from lamella to lamella, a construction that is often compared with plywood. This fibrillar arrangement was first analyzed by polarized light and later confirmed by electron microscopy. The exact delineation of the lamellae and the detailed arrangement of the fibrils, however, is still under debate. Fluorochrome labels are restricted to the mineralization front (see page 54) and appear as well-defined fluorescent bands.

Primary parallel-fibered bone shares most physiologic properties with woven bone. It is formed in earlier stages of bone formation and during periosteal and endosteal bone apposition. Its collagen fibrils run parallel to the surface but are not organized in a lamellar fashion. As in lamellar bone, fluorochrome administration gives a distinct bandlike labeling.

Based on the orientation of the lamellae, cortical bone matrix is subdivided into different compartments. The basic structural units[2,3] are the osteons (or haversian systems), longitudinally oriented cylindrical structures built around vascular (haversian) canals. In secondary osteons, the wall consists of concentric lamellae, whereas primary osteons are characterized by a more primitive parallel-fibered bone matrix (Fig 3-1). Along the periosteal and endosteal surfaces, appositional growth often results in packets of circumferential lamellae. Remnants of circumferential lamellae and of earlier generations of osteons occupy the remaining space as interstitial lamellae. The osteocytes within these remnants of cortical remodeling activity are often cut off from their vascular supply and die (Fig 3-2). Later, this devitalized matrix becomes highly mineralized.[4]

The trabeculae of cancellous bone are also composed of bone structural units (BSUs), ie, packets, walls, separated (or glued together) by cement lines. They also reflect local remodeling in earlier periods of growth and cancellous bone turnover (see page 66).[5,6]

Chemical Composition of Bone

Bone consists of about 65% mineral (mostly hydroxyapatite), 25% organic matrix, and 10% water. Collagen represents about 90% (dry weight) of the organic phase; the remaining 10% consists of proteoglycans of small molecular size and noncollagenous pro-

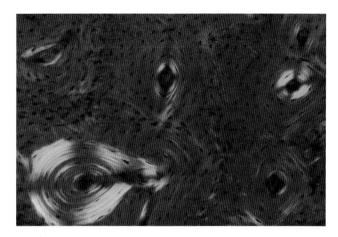

Fig 3-1 Primary and secondary osteons in equine corti-cal bone. In polarized light, secondary osteons *(bottom left)* reveal a clear-cut lamellar pattern. The wall of pri-mary osteons consists of primary parallel-fibered bone, which is less birefringent. Magnification × 125.

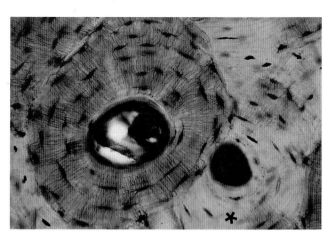

Fig 3-2 Osteons are metabolic units. Staining of osteo-cytes with basic fuchsin in undecalcified ground sections demonstrates the canalicular-lacunar system. Asterisk denotes necrotic fragment of an osteon after obliteration of the haversian canal. Magnification × 250.

teins. Among these, osteocalcin (Gla-protein) is noteworthy, since it is specific for bone. It is synthesized by osteoblasts, and its serum concentration seems to reflect bone formation.[7] Osteo-pontin is another specific component and might play a role in cell attachment, especially for osteoclasts.[8,9] Other proteins come, at least partially, from sources other than bone. Among those, osteo-nectin, a phosphorylated glycoprotein, was originally thought to link apatite to collagen.[10] The possible role of noncollagenous pro-teins in mineralization is reviewed by Boskey.[11]

Bone Cells and Bone Matrix Turnover

Osteoblasts and Bone Formation

Bone is formed by osteoblasts. These cells cover all active bone-formation sites. At regular intervals, some osteoblasts are deter-mined to become osteocytes, stop matrix extrusion on their min-eral-facing side, and become buried within the calcifying matrix by adjacent cells.[1] They maintain communication with overlying osteoblasts and neighboring osteocytes via cytoplasmic processes.

Bone formation always starts with the deposition of osteoid, which subsequently mineralizes. Woven bone is formed more rapidly than lamellar bone, and the interval between osteoid deposition and mineralization is short (1 to 3 days). The osteoid seams are small and sometimes barely visible. Woven bone often forms ridges or rods in between and around blood vessels, and thus is able to grow rapidly and to bridge gaps in a relatively

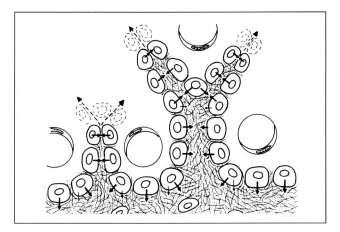

Fig 3-3 Schematic of woven bone formation illustrates bone deposition, random orientation of collagen fibrils, and osteoblast recruitment.

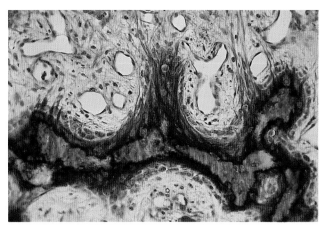

Fig 3-4 Woven bone is able to form struts and ridges. Its apposition rate depends on osteoblast recruitment. Osteoblasts are always associated with blood vessels. Goldner's trichrome stain; magnification × 100.

short time (Figs 3-3 and 3-4). The mineralization of woven bone is initiated by matrix vesicles—spherical, membrane-bound bodies with a diameter of 100 to 200 nm. They are pinched off from cytoplasmic processes (for a discussion of the role of matrix vesicles in bone and cartilage mineralization see Anderson[12]).

Compared to woven bone, lamellar bone formation takes place more slowly. The orderly deposition of collagen fibrils restricts the linear rate of osteoid production to about 1 to 2 μm per day. Lamellar bone formation requires a relatively flat surface upon which collagen fibers can be deposited in parallel and/or concentric layers. Unlike woven bone, lamellar bone is not able to construct ridges or beams. Mineralization occurs along a clearly delineated calcification (or mineralization) front that is separated from the osteoblast-bone interface by an osteoid seam (Fig 3-5). An active mineralization front exhibits some peculiar staining properties and, above all, adsorbs and permanently binds a number of substances to the rapidly growing apatite crystals. This mechanism forms the basis of labeling techniques, especially with fluorochromes, and allows accurate measurements of the mineral apposition rate (Fig 3-5). The daily linear bone apposition rate of 1 to 2 μm mentioned above was, in fact, determined at the level of the mineralization front. As long as the osteoid seams maintain a constant width, this rate is also valid for osteoid deposition. The mean thickness of osteoid is 10 μm. From this value one can derive a mineralization lag time of roughly 10 days from osteoid production to mineralization. It is not clear, however, what changes take place during the postulated maturation.

In contrast to woven bone, matrix vesicles are only rarely seen in mineralizing lamellar osteoid (Fig 3-6). To date, no structural component other than collagen has been found to be able to take over their role. Some basic requirements are considered to be

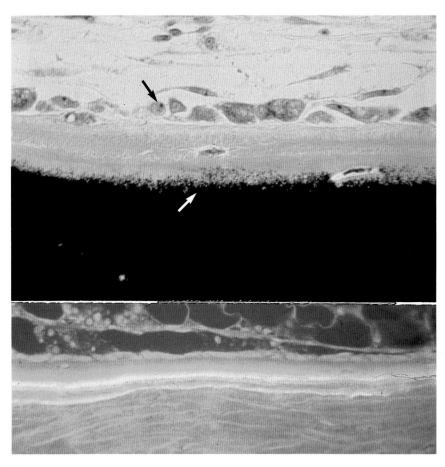

Fig 3-5 Formation of lamellar bone, human iliac crest biopsy specimen. Osteoblasts *(black arrow)*, mineralization front *(white arrow)*, osteoid seam *(between arrows)*. Von Kossa-toluidine blue stain; magnification × 800. *Below:* Fluorescence microphotograph, after double tetracycline labeling at a 1-week interval, to determine the rate of mineralization (1 to 2 µm/day).

3-5

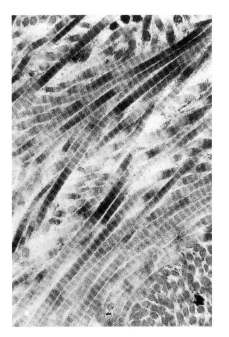

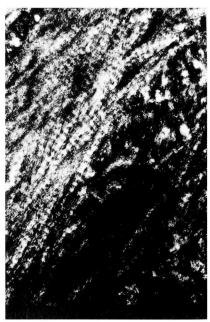

Fig 3-6 Electron micrograph of human lamellar osteoid. Magnification × 25,000.

Fig 3-7 Electron micrograph of mineralized human lamellar bone matrix. Magnification × 25,000.

3-6   3-7

compulsory for undisturbed mineralization: an adequate concentration of calcium and phosphate ions, the presence of a calcifiable matrix and nucleating agents, and the control by regulators (ie, promoters and inhibitors).[13] Collagen is a strong candidate for being a nucleator among other contenders. The mineral deposits accentuate the typical 64-nm banding pattern of collagen (Fig 3-7). In vitro tests have shown that native collagen with a 64-nm periodicity is capable of precipitating apatite in metastable solutions of calcium and phosphate ions,[14,15] although it has been postulated that this capacity depends on a combination of collagen with osteonectin[10] or phosphoproteins.[16]

Bone Lining Cells and Osteocytes: Maintenance of Bone Matrix

During bone formation, osteoblasts are entrapped as **osteocytes** in the bone matrix or they flatten out on the bone surface and transform into **bone lining cells**. The latter still belong to the osteoblast family and are called inactive or resting osteoblasts, or surface osteocytes—terms that create unnecessary confusion. It is not clear whether lining cells form a true epithelium and thus constitute a barrier between the extracellular space and the bone fluid, but they seem to control the ion exchange between these compartments. In addition, lining cells maintain cytoplasmic connections with underlying osteocytes via gap junctions between the cytoplasmic processes. The metabolic supply of osteocytes, therefore, is not only based on diffusion via the fluid in the canalicular-lacunar system, but also upon intracytoplasmic transport. Lining cells, finally, may also participate in the initiation of resorption by release of osteoclast activating factors and by active contraction, which is thought to expose the bone surface for the attachment of osteoclasts.[17]

The most conspicuous feature of osteocytes is their numerous long and delicate cytoplasmic processes extending and communicating through the canaliculi. The actual cell body is located in a somewhat larger cavity, the lacuna. The resulting canalicular-lacunar system is indispensable for cell metabolism, since a diffusion of nutrients and waste products through the heavily mineralized matrix is almost impossible. However, the transport capacity of this system has its limitations as well. The critical transport distance to keep the osteocytes alive is, in mammals, approximately 100 μm.[18] This explains why the wall thickness of osteons, as well as the wall thickness of packets in trabecular bone, seldom exceeds 100 μm (0.1 mm). Bone structural units, therefore, are not only structural, but metabolic units as well (see Fig 3-2).

Besides maintaining the integrity of the surrounding matrix, osteocytes and lining cells participate in the calcium homeostasis of the body fluids. Within the physiologic range, this activity leaves behind no visible structural traces, mainly because it takes place along an enormously extended interface between bone and osteocytes. Frost[19] and others estimate that within 1 mm^3 of lamellar bone, the surface area of the lacunae amounts to about 25 mm^2 and the canalicular surface area to about 200 mm^2. The total surface available for calcium exchange in the human skeleton must therefore be somewhere between 300 and 500 m^2.

Osteoclasts and Bone Resorption

Osteoclasts belong to a family of giant cells specialized in the breakdown of calcified matrices (bone, dentin, enamel, calcified cartilage). They differ from other giant cells, especially from foreign-body giant cells, and are conventionally identified by their location in resorption foci, their light- and electron-microscopic structure, and a positive tartrate-resistant acid phosphatase reaction (TRAP).[20,21]

Osteoclasts were accurately described in 1873 by Kölliker.[22] Actively resorbing osteoclasts adhere to the bone surface and produce lacunar pits called Howship's lacunae. They are mobile and possibly form grooves in the bone surface resembling the tracks of bark beetles. The cell diameter varies from 30 to 100 μm and the number of nuclei from 3 to 30. The cytoplasm is acidophilic and often contains vacuoles. A perpendicular striation, sometimes mistaken for a brush border, is frequently seen on the bone-facing side.

Electron microscopy has provided relevant information regarding the cytoplasmic organization of osteoclasts (Figs 3-8a to c). A detailed description of the osteoclast-bone interface has been given by Holtrop and King.[23] The marginal area of the osteoclast (clear zone, sealing part) adheres to the mineralized surface and seals off the actual resorption chamber. In the central part, the cell surface is enlarged by numerous cytoplasmic folds forming the ruffled border. The enlarged surface membrane releases hydrogen ions for acid production. After dissolution of the mineral, the exposed collagen fibrils are digested by lysosomal and nonlysosomal enzymes (for reviews see Vaes[24] and Marks and Popoff[25]).

In contrast to osteoblasts, osteoclasts do not originate from mesenchymal cells, but rather from the hemopoietic system.[26] The precursors are probably committed granulocyte-macrophage progenitor cells.[27] In spite of many studies the pathway of osteoclast formation is still not fully understood (for review see Martin et al[28]).

The average life span and the ultimate fate of osteoclasts is still debated. Unlike mononuclear cells, they cannot be regarded as an individual living unit, but rather represent an organization that constantly replaces its members. They undergo continuous renewal by fusion with additional mononuclear precursors, and obviously can also dispose of exhausted organelles and nuclei (nuclear shedding). After the injection of tritiated thymidine into adult beagle dogs, the average life span of labeled nuclei in the

Electron micrographs of an osteoclast in a rat's tibial metaphysis. *Figs 3-8a to c*

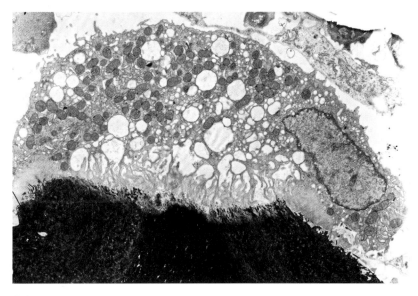

3-8a

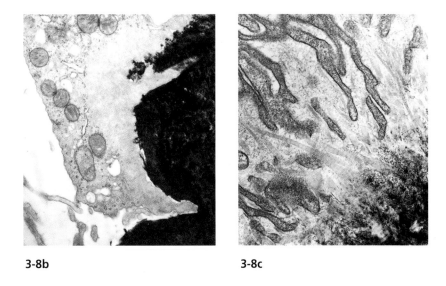

3-8b **3-8c**

Fig 3-8a The section shows only a single nuclear profile but numerous mitochondria, vesicles, and vacuoles. Magnification × 3,000.

Fig 3-8b Marginal clear zone, attachment of the cell membrane to the mineralized surface. Magnification × 7,000.

Fig 3-8c Ruffled border, signs of mineral dissolution and degradation of collagen fibrils. Magnification × 14,000.

osteoclasts was estimated to be 11 days.[29] Ultimately, osteoclasts seem to disintegrate and possibly give rise to mononuclear cells of unknown fate and potential.

Development and Growth of Bone

Prerequisites of Bone Formation

Bone formation depends on two indispensable prerequisites: **ample blood supply** and **mechanical support**. Osteoblasts function only in the immediate neighborhood of blood vessels. Reduction in oxygen seems to change their gene expression in the direction of fibrous tissue and fibrocartilage. On the other hand, the elaboration of the highly organized bone tissue requires a mechanically stable surface, and, in fact, bone is only deposited on a solid base. These principles coin the pattern of early bone development: In direct or intramembranous ossification, connective tissue serves as a template for bone deposition. During indirect or chondral ossification cartilage forms a model and, after its calcification, serves as a solid base that is first covered with, and then substituted by, bone. Endochondral ossification, as it takes place in growth cartilages, is not included in this chapter because it does not occur in defects that are not associated with a fracture, nor in fractures that heal under stable conditions (for reviews on the histophysiology of growth plates, see Schenk,[30,31] Hunziker et al,[32] and Hunziker and Schenk[33]).

Growth and Remodeling of Cortical Bone

During embryonic development, the shape of the individual bone is elaborated either directly or via a cartilaginous model. In the following fetal and postnatal growth period, the bones undergo three changes: **growth** in length and diameter, refinement of the shape by periosteal and endosteal **modeling**, and finally **remodeling** (ie, renewal and substitution of bone tissue). During these phases, the intimate relationship between bone cells and blood vessels persists, and thus these processes exert a tremendous influence on the pattern of blood supply. For this reason, the vascularity of bone is included in this chapter.

Longitudinal Growth
Endochondral ossification takes place not only in the growth plates, but also in the articular cartilages. These are responsible for the increase in size of the epiphyses and for the precise shaping of the articular surfaces, which is decisive for the congruency of synovial joints.

The growth plates separate the epiphysis from the metaphysis, and form the primary spongiosa. This comprises trabeculae with a central core of calcified cartilage. Subsequent remodeling transforms it into the secondary spongiosa, which consists solely of bone. The cortical sleeve surrounding the metaphysis is lengthened by continuous transformation of the perichondrium into periosteum and bone deposition on the newly forming parts. In many long bones, the metaphyses present a conical shape and, therefore, cause interesting modifications in the modeling pattern by the bone envelopes.

Pattern and Dynamics of Appositional Bone Growth

During growth, thickening of bones and modeling of their shape is based on formative and resorptive activities by the periosteal and endosteal envelopes. Basically, the diaphysis of a long bone grows in diameter by periosteal apposition and endosteal resorption. If apposition surpasses resorption, the cortex increases in thickness. In the adult, these activities cease and a constant cortical diameter and wall thickness are preserved. In the elderly, they resume, at least to a certain extent, and endosteal resorption may exceed periosteal apposition, resulting in an increase of the marrow cavity at the expense of the cortical thickness.

The spatial distribution of formative and resorptive activities in the periosteal and endosteal envelopes changes with the conical shaping of the metaphyses or in accordance with the modeling of curved bones. The enlargement of the thorax, specifically the growth of the ribs, provides an impressive example (Fig 3-9). With increasing length, the ribs have to displace concentrically in space, a process called cortical drift. This is achieved by periosteal apposition and endosteal resorption in the outer cortical layer and a reversed distribution of these activities in the inner cortex (Fig 3-10).

Modeling of the shape is not only regulated by the spatial distribution of formation and resorption, but by changes in the rate of apposition as well. In sites where circumferential lamellae are deposited, growth is restricted to a rate of 1 to 2 μm per day (Fig 3-11a). If a more rapid growth is required, a composite of woven and lamellar bone is deposited, resulting in the formation of primary osteons (Fig 3-11b). Essentially, the capacity of woven bone to form crests and ridges is activated in order to produce grooves and, later on, tunnels around longitudinally oriented blood vessels. Subsequently, the tunnels are narrowed by the deposition of concentric layers until the primary osteons are completed. This mechanism results in a manyfold increase of the daily apposition, mainly because the growth of woven bone does not depend on the rate of matrix formation, but rather on the recruitment and proliferation of new osteoblasts.

Vascular Supply of Primary Osteons

The vessels incorporated in primary osteons emanate from the envelope engaged in their formation. For the most part, they remain connected to their source, although, in deeper layers, there are always numerous anastomoses with the vascular net

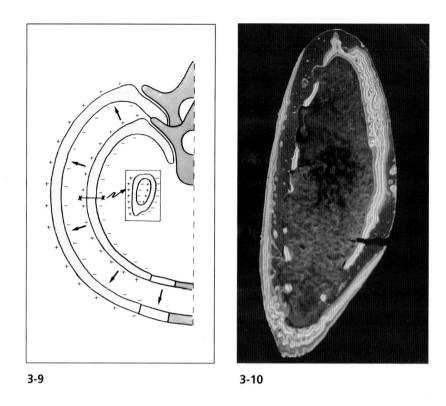

3-9   3-10

Fig 3-9   Cortical drift. Schematic of spatial dislocation with growth and cross-sectional distribution of formation (+) and resorption (–).

Fig 3-10   Sequential fluorochrome labeling in a rabbit's rib over 8 weeks confirms the growth pattern illustrated in Fig 3-9. (Specimen and micrograph courtesy of Professor B. Rahn.)

Appositional growth pattern by the periosteal envelope in a canine tibia. Polychrome fluorescent labeling at weekly intervals over 8 weeks.

Figs 3-11a and b

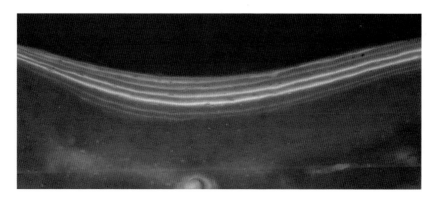

3-11a

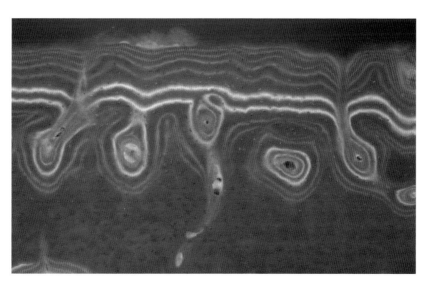

3-11b

Fig 3-11a Strictly lamellar bone deposition leads to formation of circumferential lamellae. Magnification × 120.

Fig 3-11b Woven bone formation results in ridges that fuse around blood vessels and give rise to primary osteons. Observe the net gain in periosteal apposition rate. Magnification × 120.

originating from the opposite envelope. Since periosteal growth far outweighs endosteal apposition, stripping of the periosteum or rupture and compression by surgical devices predictably creates avascular zones in the outer layer of compact bone.

Cortical Remodeling: Formation of Secondary Osteons

Primary osteons are formed during appositional growth whereas secondary osteons result from substitution, which is initiated by resorption followed by formation. The remodeling sequence was originally studied in transverse sections (Figs 3-12a to c). First, a resorption canal is formed by osteoclasts. Later, osteoblasts appear and start refilling this canal with concentric lamellae. In compact human bone, completed secondary osteons have an outer diameter of 200 to 250 μm, the vascular canal measuring 50 to 80 μm. The wall thickness reaches 70 to 100 μm[34] and varies somewhat with age.[35] Secondary osteons run parallel to the long axis of the bone. Their length is difficult to measure because of frequent branching. As a coherent cylindrical structure they are seldom more than 2 to 3 mm long and are interconnected by transverse vascular channels (Volkmann's canals) at intervals of 0.5 to 1.0 mm.

Secondary osteons are always separated from the surrounding matrix by a cement line. Two types of cement lines are distinguished: arresting lines and reversal lines. Arresting lines are smooth and strictly parallel to the lamellae. They appear when bone formation is arrested and, after a resting period, resumes again. Reversal lines are formed when resorption is terminated and then followed by osteoblastic bone deposition. Howship's lacunae left behind by the osteoclasts give them a crenated appearance (Fig 3-12c).

Longitudinal sections of newly forming osteons have shown that bone resorption and formation are coupled in space and time, and occur in discrete remodeling sites called "bone-metabolizing units" or BMUs (originally bone multicellular unit[2,3]). Within the tip of a resorption canal, osteoclasts are assembled in a cutter cone (Fig 3-13). The osteoclasts advance longitudinally and simultaneously widen the resorption canal up to its final diameter. The tip of a vascular loop follows immediately behind the osteoclasts. This loop lies in the center of the canal and is surrounded by perivascular cells, including osteoclast and osteoblast precursors. Behind the osteoclasts, the wall of the canals is lined by mononuclear cells, but only for a short distance of 100 to 200 μm, corresponding to a reversal phase of 1 to 2 days. Then osteoblasts appear and deposit lamellar osteoid, which will mineralize 8 to 10 days later. In the longitudinally advancing system, the canal assumes a conical shape (closing cone). Completion of the osteon requires, depending on the species, 2 to 4 months. These measurements and calculations are based on sequential fluorochrome labeling (Fig 3-14) and also allow an accurate determination of the osteoclastic resorption rate in longitudinal sections, which amounts to 50 to 60 μm/day in dogs.[36–38]

Cortical bone remodeling in the humerus of an adult man; transverse sections through evolving secondary osteons.

Figs 3-12a to c

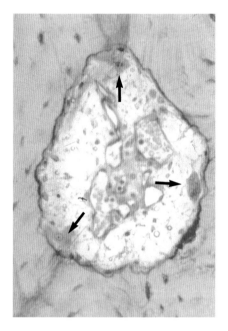

3-12a

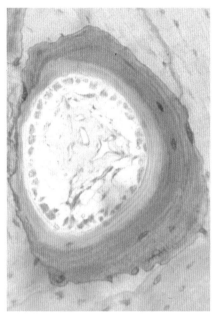

3-12b

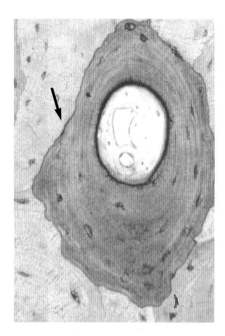

3-12c

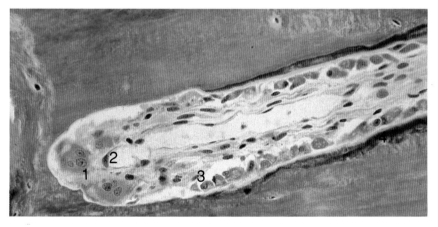

3-13

Fig 3-12a   Resorption canal with osteoclasts *(arrows)*.

Fig 3-12b   Osteoblasts deposit concentric lamellae.

Fig 3-12c   Completed secondary osteon, bound by a cement line *(arrow)*. Figs 12a to c toluidine blue surface stain; magnification × 240.

Fig 3-13   Longitudinal section through the tip of an evolving secondary osteon (BMU) during fracture repair in a canine radius. Microtome section, Goldner's trichrome, magnification × 160. (1) Osteoclastic cutter cone, (2) vascular loop, (3) osteoblasts, (4) osteoid seam.

Fig 3-14   Sequential polychrome labeling of a BMU at weekly intervals *(arrowheads)* to measure the daily osteoclastic resorption rate.

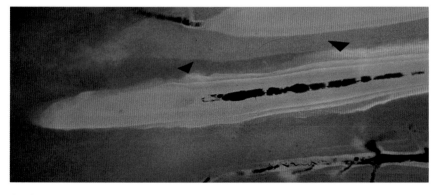

3-14

Vascular Supply of Secondary Osteons

In the diaphysis of long bones, formation of secondary osteons usually starts near the endosteal surface and gradually progresses toward the periosteum. As a result, the rule of thumb that the inner two thirds of the cortex is connected to the medullary circulation and the outer third to periosteal vessels[39] is generally accepted, although it is subjected to frequent local variations.

Formation and Remodeling of Cancellous Bone

Development and Growth

Early in embryonic development, a primary spongework of trabeculae appears as condensation in the mesenchyme, always in the vicinity of blood vessels. This intramembranous ossification mainly takes place in the head. In the viscerocranium, it results in the formation of the premaxilla, maxilla, palatine, nasal, lacrimal, zygomatic, tympanic bone, and the vomer. The mandible, as well, forms directly in the mesenchyme, lateral to Meckel's cartilage. Later, a secondary cartilage appears on the future capitulum of the condylar process. This cartilage contributes to the growth of the collum by endochondral ossification and finally differentiates into articular cartilage.

In long bones, cancellous bone arises from the growth plate in the metaphysis. In the epiphyses it is initially formed in secondary ossification centers and later completed by endochondral ossification from articular cartilage. During growth, the cancellous bone is thoroughly remodeled or eliminated by the expansion of the marrow cavity.

Modeling and Functional Adaptation of Cancellous Bone

Modeling and remodeling continues after cessation of growth. Microscopically, an astonishingly high number of cement lines, both of the arresting and reversal types, indicate an intensive turnover. As mentioned earlier, modeling indicates a change in shape, whereas remodeling means tissue replacement or substitution. Modeling in the spongiosa specifically changes the architecture of the cancellous bone. In fact, the architecture of the trabecular framework is originally determined by the growth pattern. Later, it undergoes profound changes that result in a structural adaptation to the prevailing functional load, or, as often stated, "according to Wolff's law."[40] This adaptation enables bone to withstand a given stress with a minimum amount of material. This saves weight and conserves metabolic energy. The mechanism of functional adaptation is not, by any means, fully understood, and at present Wolff's law just offers a convenient way to accept it as a fact, without being forced to look for other explanations.

Trabecular Bone Remodeling

In contrast to the concept of modeling, remodeling means substitution of bone tissue without a change in architecture. This improves the quality of the tissue, both in view of its mechanical as well as its metabolic properties. Remodeling replaces discrete portions (or packets) with new lamellar bone (Figs 3-15a to c). Formation of a new packet begins with a local recruitment of osteoclasts that form a cavity on the trabecular surface. The mean depth of these cavities is around 50 µm and rarely exceeds 70 µm. At the end of this **resorptive phase**, the osteoclasts move on or disappear, and after a short intermission or **reversal phase**, osteoblasts start depositing new bone **(formative phase)**. The completed new packet is again confined by a cement (reversal) line. In analogy to the osteons, it is considered a "bone structural unit" (BSU), and the cell population involved in its formation a BMU. In view of the extent of the trabecular surface in the human skeleton, the control and dynamics of cancellous bone remodeling play an important role in the pathogenesis of metabolic bone disease, particularly in osteoporosis.

Regulation of Bone Remodeling

Systemically, bone remodeling is activated by growth hormone and thyroid and parathyroid hormones, and inhibited by calcitonin and cortisone. Locally, bone remodeling is activated by any trauma to the bone, ie, fractures, surgical devices, or implant insertion. A temporary interruption of the blood supply with associated devitalization and necrosis of bone tissue results in substantial activation of remodeling, even without any concomitant mechanical lesion. It triggers revascularization and substitution of necrotic zones by vital tissue.

The coupling phenomenon is of special interest because it involves cells of rather different origin in both cortical and trabecular remodeling units. This has stimulated the search for coupling factors,[41,42] but the initiation of the coupled resorptive and formative activities is obviously based on a concerted action of multiple factors engaged in osteoclast activation, osteoblast proliferation and differentiation, matrix formation, and mineralization. In addition, the concept of coupling is not only related to the coordination of specific cellular activities, but also suggests that their performance should be balanced in order to replace a certain volume of resorbed bone by the same amount of newly formed tissue.[32,43]

Trabecular bone remodeling in a human iliac crest biopsy.
Figs 3-15a to c

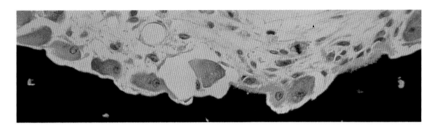

3-15a

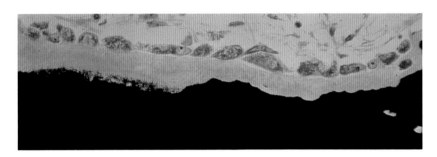

3-15b

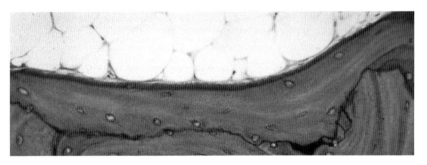

3-15c

Fig 3-15a   Resorptive phase. Von Kossa-McNeal stain; magnification × 320.

Fig 3-15b   Early formative phase. Von Kossa-McNeal stain; magnification × 320.

Fig 3-15c   Newly formed packet (BSU), clearly delineated by a reversal line. Surface staining with toluidine blue; magnification × 200.

Biology of Bone Regeneration

Regeneration is commonly understood as replacement of vanishing or lost components in the body by equally highly organized elements. Many tissues or organ systems undergo a **physiologic regeneration**, ie, a continuous replacement of cells or tissue elements. Blood cells, epithelia, glands, or the endometrium during the reproductive cycle are the best-known examples. Nerve cells and muscle fibers, on the other hand, cannot proliferate. Remodeling of cortical and trabecular bone also represents regeneration; not only are cells replaced, but also matrix. In adult articular cartilage, on the contrary, chondrocytes only rarely undergo mitotic division, and the turnover of matrix components is extremely slow.

Reparative regeneration takes place when tissues are lost because of injury or disease. Supporting tissues have differing repair capacities. Articular cartilage is practically unable to regenerate, and full-thickness defects are filled by fibrous tissue or replaced by less differentiated fibrocartilage. Fibrous connective tissue appears superficially to possess a good capacity for repair. However, highly differentiated connective tissues, like ligaments and tendons, will never reach the original level of organization and will heal with a scar of reduced mechanical strength. Bone has the unique potential to restore its original structure completely, but there are certain limitations. The reconstruction of the original level of organization occurs sequentially and closely repeats the pattern of bone development and growth. Likewise, some basic conditions have to be ensured, such as ample blood supply and mechanical stability, provided by a solid base. This pattern of bone regeneration and some possibilities to promote and to protect the repair process will be demonstrated by histologic observations in selected experimental studies.

Activation of Bone Regeneration

Any bone lesion (fracture, defect, insertion of implants, interruption of blood supply) activates local bone regeneration by the release of growth factors (GF) and inductors. Bone is, in fact, one of the richest sources for growth factors. Among the growth factors detected in bone, some are produced by bone cells (insulin-like growth factor [IGF], transforming growth factor [TGF], fibroblast growth factor [FGF], platelet-derived growth factor [PDGF]) whereas others are synthesized by bone-related tissues (interleukin-1 [IL-1], tumor necrosis factor a [TNFa]). In addition, some **bone inducing factors** are of great interest, such as Lacroix's osteogenin[44] and the bone morphogenetic protein (BMP) of Urist et al,[45,46] which has now been fractionated into at least seven different proteins (BMP family[47]).

Osteoinduction in its classical concept implies initiation of heterotopic bone formation (in sites where bone physiologically does not normally exist). It is, however, just as frequently applied if ossification is activated in contact with existing bones, ie, in the case of orthotopic bone induction. A concept that helps to clarify the situation was proposed by Friedenstein,[48,49] who distinguished between determined and inducible osteoprecursor cells. Determined osteoprecursor cells are found in tissues in direct vicinity to bone, such as bone marrow stroma cells, and cells in the periosteum, endosteum, and intracortical canals. These cells react to induction with proliferation and differentiate directly into osteoblasts. Inducible osteoprecursor cells are found far from bone. These fibroblastlike cells are abundant in subcutaneous connective tissue, skeletal muscles, and the spleen and kidney capsule. Their reaction to inductive stimuli (such as BMP) is more complex and, in fact, mimics endochondral bone formation.[50] After subcutaneous implantation in rats, proliferation of mesenchymal cells starts after 3 to 4 days. From day 5 to 8 on, cartilage develops and, within one day, starts to mineralize. Vascular invasion and bony substitution of the calcifying cartilage follows from day 10 to 11 on. Intermediate cartilage differentiation seems to be mandatory if induction acts on inducible osteoprecursor cells. The response is always indirect bone formation.

In orthotopic bone induction, the inducing principle acts on determined osteoprecursor cells, and the reaction is direct bone formation. The lag phase is short, seldom longer than 1 to 3 days, and the newly formed bone is laid down on pre-existing bone surfaces. It is questionable whether one should call this process bone induction or just activation or stimulation of bone formation and, furthermore, whether the same or different compounds are involved in its initiation. The whole cascade of events that is triggered by the numerous growth factors is still unclear. However, it is clear that only some BMPs and other members of the TGFβ superfamily are able to induce heterotopic bone formation. In the context of bone repair and bone regeneration, use of the term *activation* for the orthotopic induction of bone formation is therefore preferred.

Repair of Bone Defects

The repair of bone defects is a good model for the study of bone regeneration. In contrast to fractures, defects are less subject to mechanical factors and to obstructions of the blood supply. Defect healing, therefore, has been used in many classical experiments dealing with the influence of surgical and pharmacologic measures to improve bone regeneration. The basic pattern of defect healing in relation to physiologic ossification and growth is discussed below.

Repair of Small Cortical Defects

Within the scope of experiments dealing with primary or direct fracture healing,[31] Johner[51] examined the healing of bore holes with diameters between 0.1 and 1.0 mm in the tibia of rabbits. Bone formation within these holes starts within a couple of days, without preceding osteoclastic resorption, and reveals a clearcut size dependency. Holes with a diameter in the range of osteons (0.2 mm) are concentrically filled with lamellar bone (Figs 3-16a and b). In larger holes, a scaffold of woven bone is formed and then lamellar bone is deposited in the newly formed intertrabecular spaces, which have a corresponding diameter of 150 to 200 μm (Figs 3-17a and b). As in appositional growth (page 59), lamellar bone deposition is restricted by its appositional rate to a couple of microns per day, whereas woven bone rapidly bridges larger defects. After 4 weeks, both the small and the larger defects are filled by compact bone. There is, however, a threshold for this rapid bridging by woven bone. This threshold lies around 1 mm for bore holes in rabbit cortical bone.[52] Experimental studies on bony ingrowth into porous acetabular components for total hips in dogs demonstrate similar results, summarized in the often quoted catchword "osteogenic jumping distance." It indicates that bone is not able to cross gaps wider than 1 mm by one single jump.[53] In the case of implants, the situation becomes even more difficult because bridging the defect starts from the bony side only. This does not mean that larger holes or gaps will stay open indefinitely, but filling takes longer, and there is no doubt that bore holes of 3 to 5 mm (eg, holes after screw removal) persist for several weeks if not months until repair is completed.

Completion of filling, however, does not mean termination of healing. The bony regenerate appears compact, but its structure is still far from the appearance of the osteonal cortical bone. Osteonal cortical bone must be formed by haversian remodeling. Remodeling starts in the cortex immediately surrounding the hole about 3 weeks after creation of the defect. Remodeling is activated by the local tissue and vascular damage produced by drilling. From the margin of the defect it progresses into the newly formed bone and replaces it by longitudinally oriented, secondary osteons (Figs 3-18a and b). Within a couple of months, the small cortical defects are fully reconstructed and can only be identified by detailed microscopic evaluation.

In summary, repair of small cortical defects can be divided into two phases that closely resemble the formation of compact bone during development and growth. The simple lesion produced by drilling a hole seems to activate a programmed sequence of events, which starts filling the defect by appositional bone formation (page 59) and then leads to a structural integration of the defect area by haversian remodeling (page 62).

Repair of small cortical defects. Bur holes in the cortex of rabbit's tibiae, 0.2-mm diameter.

Figs 3-16a and b

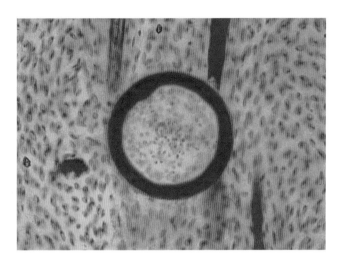

Fig 3-16a After 1 week.

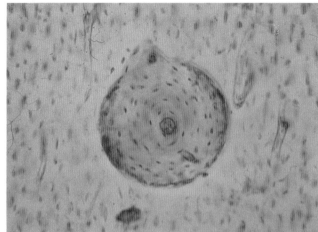

Fig 3-16b After 4 weeks.

Bur holes with 0.4-mm diameter. Basic fuchsin stain.

Figs 3-17a and b

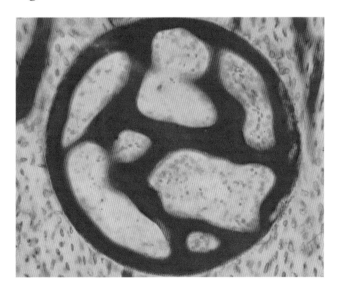

Fig 3-17a After 1 week.

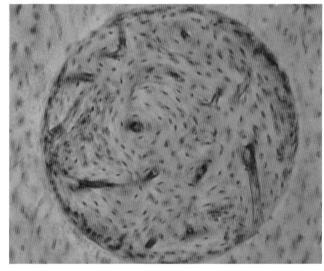

Fig 3-17b After 4 weeks.

Microradiographs of repair of small cortical defect, haversian remodeling. *Figs 3-18a and b*

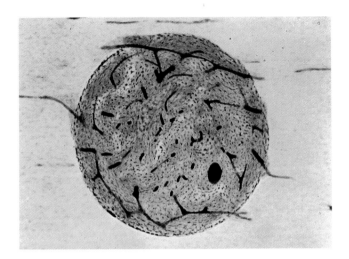

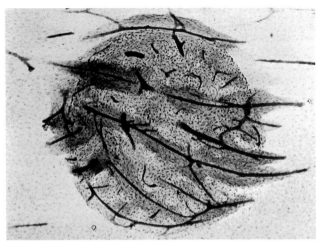

Fig 3-18a A 0.6-mm hole after 6 weeks.

Fig 3-18b After 6 months, the original compact filling is partially substituted by newly formed osteons.

Repair of Small Cancellous Bone Defects

Small cancellous bone defects reveal a similar healing pattern. Healing also occurs in two phases, starting with woven bone formation across the defect and within the adjacent intertrabecular spaces. This primary scaffold is then reinforced by concentric filling of the spongework lattice by primary parallel-fibered bone, which increases considerably the density in the former defect area. In a second phase, remodeling restores the trabecular architecture.

Histology of Direct Fracture Healing

Although fracture repair is not covered in this chapter, the striking similarity of defect repair and direct or primary fracture healing has to be mentioned. It is the logical consequence of exact anatomic reduction of the fracture and the consecutive reduction of the size of the interfragmentary gaps, and rigid fixation, which provides stable mechanical conditions as in a defect site.[31]

Promotion of Bone Regeneration

As outlined before, bone tissue exhibits an astonishing regenerative potential and perfectly restores its original structure and its mechanical properties. But this capacity has its limits and may even fail if certain conditions are not fulfilled. Factors that impede or prevent bone repair are, among others: *(1)* failure of vascularity, *(2)* mechanical instability, *(3)* oversized defects, and *(4)* competing tissues of high proliferative activity.

Failure of vascularity and instability are commonly associated with fractures, and often result in nonunions. Instability causes hypertrophic nonunions with abundant callus formation and differentiation of fibrocartilage in the fracture gap. Persisting instability arrests endochondral ossification by inhibition of fibrocartilage mineralization.[31] Interruption of the blood supply causes necrosis of fragments or fragment ends and impairs bone union. Loss of fragments or surgical removal of necrotic fragments creates defects that are often too large to be filled by bone spontaneously. Finally, the cells in neighboring soft tissues might proliferate more rapidly and occupy the defect site faster than bone can grow.

In fact, fibrous connective tissue regenerates faster than more highly differentiated tissue. This leads to scar formation at the site of the lesion. To a certain extent, bone regeneration can compete with fibrous tissue and, moreover, is able to replace the initially formed fibrous tissue at a later time, at least partially. In addition, there are means to promote and to support bone regeneration. In the following paragraphs, the principle of such methods is discussed in the light of some experimental observations.

Osteoconduction

Bony filling of larger defects is greatly facilitated by osteoconduction, ie, by offering a framework or scaffold as a template and enlarged solid base for bone deposition. Certain conditions must be fulfilled for successful osteoconduction: *(1)* the scaffold must consist of a bioinert or bioactive material, and *(2)* the shape and dimensions of its external and internal structure should favor tissue ingrowth and bone deposition. Ideally, the material should be replaceable by bone. This is only possible if it can be resorbed and substituted during the remodeling phase of bone repair.

As far as tissue compatibility is concerned, both bioinert and bioactive compounds allow a direct deposition of bone on their surfaces. By definition, only a bioactive material establishes a chemical bond and thus a firm attachment to bone. In view of shape and dimensions, spongious bone provides the ideal conditions for bony ingrowth, namely an overall volume density of 20%

to 30% (equal to a porosity of 70% to 80%), a mean diameter of plates or rods of approximately 200 μm, an average intertrabecular pore size of approximately 500 μm, and ample pore interconnections. How osteoconduction can promote bone repair is demonstrated by a few selected examples of bone grafts and bone substitutes.

Incorporation and Integration of Cancellous Bone Grafts

Cancellous autografts set the standard for judging the benefits of osteoconduction because there is no risk of any immunologic reaction; a prompt transplantation keeps many cells alive. The incorporation and integration of autologous cancellous bone is well known and is demonstrated here by means of histologic observations of equine metacarpal and metatarsal bones. In these experiments (performed in collaboration with an equine surgeon, Professor Björn von Salis, Frauenfeld, Switzerland) cortical bur holes with diameters of approximately 5 mm were filled with tightly fitting cancellous bone cylinders, and empty holes served as controls. By 4 months, the empty holes were incompletely filled by new bone, which was deposited on the surrounding walls, leaving the center free (Fig 3-19). A cancellous graft divided the defect into smaller compartments (Fig 3-20), and these were completely filled with new bone by 4 months as well (Fig 3-21). The new bone was bound firmly to the surface of the grafted bone, the interface being marked by a regular cement line. With other methods, eg, microradiography, the graft remained clearly identifiable within the almost compact bony regenerate by its higher mineral density (Fig 3-21). The graft's contours were also traced using fluorochrome labels given during the first period of bony incorporation (Fig 3-22). The structure of the compact bony regenerate did not yet correspond to the surrounding osteonal bone. During the following months it underwent extensive haversian remodeling. As a result, the primary regenerate, together with the grafted scaffold, was almost completely replaced, and because fluorochrome labeling was discontinued after 4 months, the labeled areas disappeared (Fig 3-23). In the eighth and ninth months, two more labels were given. These labels were located in newly forming osteons (BMUs) and appeared in the fluorescent photomicrographs as small circular profiles (Fig 3-23).

Incorporation and integration of cancellous autografts, therefore, reveal the same pattern as defect repair (page 69), provided that the grafted area itself exhibits the necessary osteogenetic potential and fulfills the other requirements for bone formation, such as good vascularity and mechanical stability.

Incorporation and Integration of Allografts and Bone Substitutes

Allografts, as well as some bone-derived or synthetic bone substitutes, have similar osteoconductive properties. However, degrada-

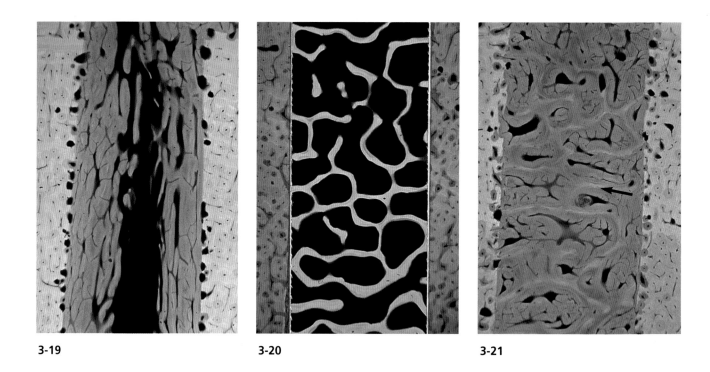

3-19   3-20   3-21

Fig 3-19 Osteoconduction. Incorporation of cancellous bone grafts in cortical bur holes in equine metatarsal bones. Incomplete bony filling of a 4-mm control hole after 4 months. Microradiograph; magnification × 8.

Fig 3-20 Fotomontage showing subdivision of the defect space by insertion of a cancellous bone cylinder.

Fig 3-21 Bony filling of the intertrabecular space of a cancellous autograft after 4 months, the grafted spongiosa still being recognizable in the microradiograph by its higher mineral density *(arrow)*. Magnification × 8.

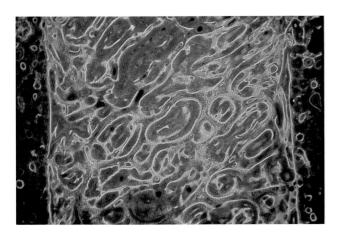

3-22

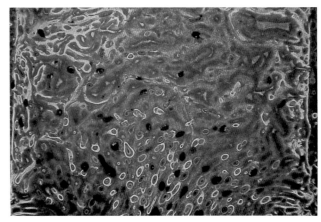

3-23

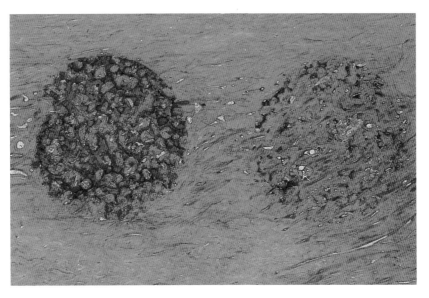

3-24

Fig 3-22 Osteoconduction. Cancellous autograft after 4 months. Fluorochrome labels given in the third and fourth months outline the contour of the spongiosa in the inserted cylinder with a diameter of 6 mm. Magnification × 10.

Fig 3-23 Integration of cancellous bone grafts in equine metatarsal bone by haversian remodeling after 10 months. Fluorescence microscopy; Magnification × 10.

Fig 3-24 Osteoconduction. Incorporation and integration of porous calcium phosphate ceramics in a canine tibia after 21 months. *Left:* A 5-mm hydroxyapatite cylinder (CEROS 80) showing bony filling of the pores. *Right:* A tricalcium phosphate cylinder (CEROS 82) of identical initial structure underwent extensive haversian remodeling and substitution within the same period. Magnification × 8.

tion and substitution by viable bone is often poor. If the implanted material is not resorbable—as in the case of certain porous hydroxyapatite implants—the incorporation is restricted to bone apposition to the material surface, but no substitution occurs during the remodeling phase (Fig 3-24). Resorbable tricalcium phosphate ceramics (tricalcium phosphate) of identical initial structure undergo resorption and extensive substitution under the same experimental conditions.[55] In view of mechanical properties, however, cancellous bone grafts still clearly surpass all bone-derived, natural (coral), or synthetic porous substitutes.

In the treatment of extensive defects, however, autografts also have restrictions, mainly because of limited availability. Microvascular, corticospongious transplants are technically demanding and often do not reconstruct a full-sized substitute. In such conditions, callus distraction, as developed by Ilizarov[56,57] since 1965, has become a successful and biologically interesting alternative.

Distraction Osteogenesis (Callus Distraction)

Historically, lengthening of bones by stretching callus in its early stages of formation goes back to the last century.[58] Ilizarov[56,57] has systematically studied and perfected this principle, which now has gained worldwide recognition and application for bone lengthening and, even more important, for bridging diaphyseal defects in long bones by segment transport.

From 5 to 8 days after performing an osteotomy or corticotomy, the callus forming in the osteotomy gap is stretched at a rate of about 1 mm/day in four or more increments. Stabilization and distraction is achieved by more or less complicated (and not always comfortable) external fixators. The importance of stability has been experimentally demonstrated by Ilizarov. Micromovements (other than the controlled daily distraction) inevitably lead to nonunion of the fibrous type, or cartilage formation and delayed and incomplete bone formation.[57] Careful protection of the vascular supply of both the transported segment and the tissue within the gap is another, decisive prerequisite for the success of the procedure.

Bone formation within the gradually extending gap is monitored by radiographs. Calcification appears by 2 to 4 weeks, starting from both fragment ends toward a radiolucent intermediate zone, also referred to as a fibrous interzone or growth zone. The newly formed bone has a stringy appearance, suggesting the formation of thin longitudinal rods and plates. Its longitudinal growth rate is surprisingly high. As long as it keeps pace with distraction, it amounts to almost 500 μm (half a millimeter) a day and one can expect that, within a month, a newly created space of almost 1 inch is filled with a bony regenerate. The density of this bone tissue, however, is low, and it takes months for its corticalization, and possibly years for reconstruction of a true cortex via haversian remodeling. Weight bearing, under the protection of the fixation device, can start much earlier, and the removal of the fixator is also recommended long before completion of remodeling.

The histology of callus distraction has been described in experimental animals[59,60] and in humans.[61] The fibrous interzone is the center of growth, where neoangiogenesis and proliferation of fibroblasts takes place. The continuous stretching aligns the collagen into longitudinal fiber bundles and, correspondingly, the vessels extend into the interfibrillar spaces. Starting from the surfaces of the bone ends, woven bone grows into the longitudinally oriented fibrovascular compartments, initially as thin rods or plates; these increase in thickness and fuse to plates surrounding the blood vessels (Fig 3-25). The collagen fibers can be described as a trellis. The bony spicules that climb along these fiber bundles are lengthened by bone deposition on their tips, accomplished by newly recruited osteoblasts (Fig 3-26). The longitudinal growth rate, therefore, depends on proliferation and differentiation of osteoblast precursors, whereas the bone apposition rate determines the daily increase in width of the individual trabeculae. The resulting primary scaffold consists of woven bone, which is later reinforced by lamellar bone, and finally reorganized by haversian remodeling, strictly according to the rules that govern appositional growth and remodeling of the cortex (page 59), or the repair of small cortical defects (page 69).

In addition to the impressive performance of callus distraction, some mention must be made of the side effects that have been reported in the literature. These include rupture of blood vessels, leading to local hematoma, or microfractures in newly formed trabeculae, which usually heal by microcallus formation.[61] Furthermore, extensive limb lengthening may cause complications related to overstretching of other tissue (muscle, tendon, nerves, blood vessels).

Guided Bone Regeneration

The use of barrier membranes to facilitate bone healing was originally developed by Hurley[62] and Boyne[63] (see chapter 2 in this book).

Later, barrier membranes were applied for promotion of periodontal regeneration.[64] The method was then tested in different types of bone defects and around dental implants, both experimentally and clinically.[65–70]

Guided bone regeneration (GBR) refers more precisely to the goal of the membrane application than guided tissue regeneration. However, it may inappropriately recall the principle of osteoconduction, ie, the provision of a scaffold that serves as a base for bone deposition. This is not the case. Guided bone regeneration promotes bone formation by protection against an invasion of competing, nonosteogenic tissues. To this end, bone defects are tightly covered by a barrier membrane of defined permeability and

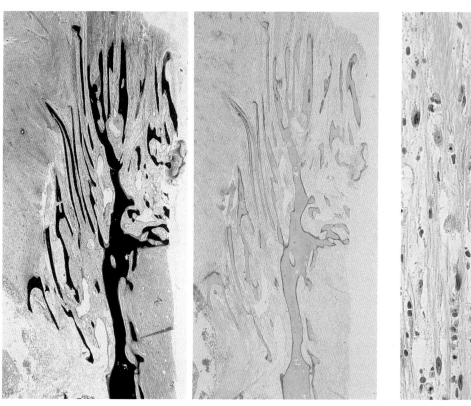

3-25

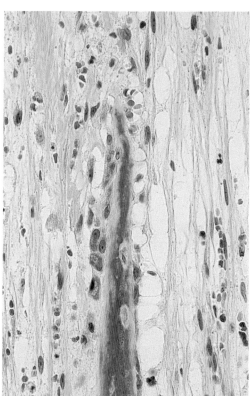

3-26

Fig 3-25 Distraction osteogenesis. Longitudinal section of a superficial (subperiosteal) biopsy after completion of a 25-mm bone lengthening in a human femur. Note the parallel alignment of tiny bony spicules growing from the fragment ends upward into the fibrous interzone. *Left:* von Kossa-McNeal stain. *Right:* Goldner stain. Magnification × 5.

Fig 3-26 Tip of a bony spicule, advancing into the longitudinal compartment provided by the stretched collagen fibers. Magnification × 300.

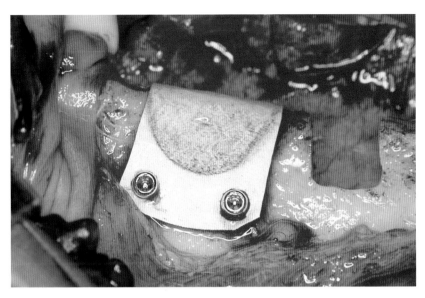

Fig 3-27 Guided bone regeneration surgical procedure. Exposure of the alveolar crest in a canine mandible, 2 months after extraction of premolar teeth. The distal defect is open; the mesial is covered with a barrier membrane. Miniscrews fix the membrane and mark the corners of the defect for radiography.

excellent tissue compatibility. Both resorbable and nonresorbable membranes are currently under investigation, as are membranes with different porosity and modified mechanical properties.

Following are histologic observations of GBR, gained from an experimental study in the canine mandible using expanded poly-tetrafluoroethylene (e-PTFE) membranes.[71]

Surgical Procedure

Four foxhound dogs were used in the experiments. Two months before surgery, the mandibular premolar teeth were extracted and the sockets were allowed to heal. After exposure of the alveolar crest, two defects (approximately 8 mm deep and 12 to 15 mm long) were created on each side of the mandible (Fig 3-27). The e-PTFE membranes were cut to the appropriate size, placed over the defect area, and adapted as closely as possible to the surrounding bone surface. Their position was secured by two miniscrews, placed below the corners of the defect in the buccal wall. Two types of membranes were implanted: a commercially available e-PTFE membrane designed for alveolar ridge GBR and, as a modification, an e-PTFE membrane reinforced by polypropylene mesh. Intravenously aspired blood was injected underneath the membranes to remove air and to ensure formation of a homogeneous blood clot.

Control defects were not covered with membranes. Miniscrews were also inserted in analogous positions near the control defects to facilitate orientation in the radiographs.

Histologic Preparation

Two dogs were sacrificed after 2 months and the other two at 4 months. The specimens were removed and fixed in 10% neutral formalin. The blocks were embedded without decalcification in methylmethacrylate. Coronal (buccolingual) sections were cut with a diamond wafer blade, glued on Plexiglas plates, ground and polished on carborundum paper, and finally surface stained with toluidine blue or toluidine blue and basic fuchsin. Selected parts of the ground sections were later cut on a microtome and stained with Goldner's trichrome or by the methods of von Kossa-McNeal, as described in Schenk et al.[72]

Microscopic Examination

To facilitate description, the following terms are used for topographic orientation. Lateral view of defect or regenerate: mesial/middle/distal portion; mesial or distal wall; roof or bottom. Coronal = buccolingual sectional plane: periphery or center (peripheral, central); roof or bottom; inside or outside of membrane; inner or outer compartment.

Healing of Control Defects

Control defects show a consistent repair pattern: Bone formation is restricted to the margins of the defect, where bony covers develop that close the surgically opened marrow space in the bottom as well as in the mesial and distal walls (Figs 3-28 and 3-29). Closure of the marrow space is completed after 2 months, but bone formation makes no further progress and a deep indentation persists in the mandibular crest (Fig 3-30). At 4 months the situation remains virtually unchanged, except for some increase in density. The volume of new bone covering the marrow cavity does not increase significantly.

Healing Underneath Barrier Membranes

Membrane protection results in a dramatic change in bone and tissue regeneration. The membrane maintains the space created during surgery and clearly separates the outer, gingival compartment from the inner space, which is mainly accessible from the marrow cavity (Fig 3-31).

This inner compartment is initially occupied by a blood clot, and by 2 months remnants of the coagulum can still be recognized in the middle portion of the defect (Figs 3-32 and 3-33). The hematoma, however, is completely penetrated by granulation tissue and blood vessels. The majority of the secluded volume now consists of a spongious bony regenerate that encloses, between its trabeculae, a labyrinth of tiny, interdigitating marrow spaces filled with hypervascularized, loose connective tissue. Both the vessels and the fibrous tissue are in continuity with the original bone marrow. Bone formation starts, as in the controls, from the margins of the defect and first spreads over the openings of the marrow cavity (Fig 3-34). From these covers it further expands into

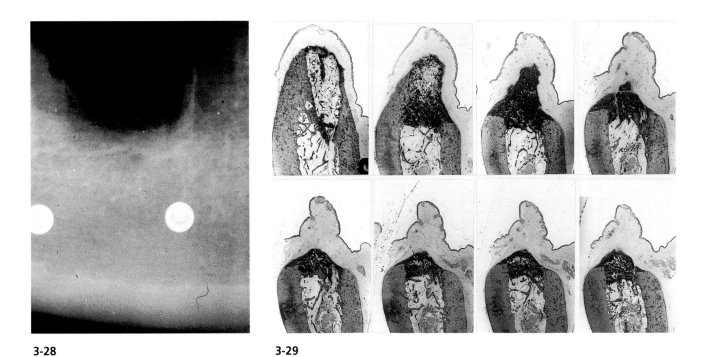

3-28   3-29

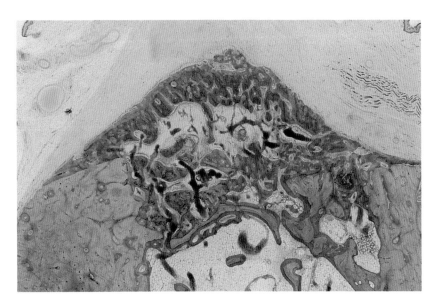

3-30

Fig 3-28   Control defect, 2-month postoperative radiograph. Bone formation is restricted to the margins of the defects. (Reproduced with permission from Schenk et al.[71])

Fig 3-29   Serial sections at steps of 1.5 mm, starting from the medial margin *(left in Fig 3-28)* into the middle portion. Magnification × 1.2. (Reproduced with permission from Schenk et al.[71])

Fig 3-30   Section through the middle portion of a control defect after 2 months. A bony cover seals the marrow space in the bottom of the defect. Magnification × 12.

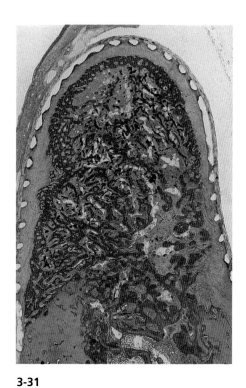

3-31

Fig 3-31 Buccolingual section of a membrane-covered defect after 2 months shows the bony filling of the secluded volume beneath the membrane. Surface staining with toluidine blue and basic fuchsin; magnification × 4.

Fig 3-32 Radiograph of a membrane-covered defect after 2 months shows bony ingrowth from the mesial and distal wall, as well as from the bottom. (Reproduced with permission from Schenk et al.[71])

Fig 3-33 Selected buccolingual sections of a membrane-covered defect after 2 months, in mesial-distal sequence. Magnification × 1.2. (Reproduced with permission from Schenk et al.[71])

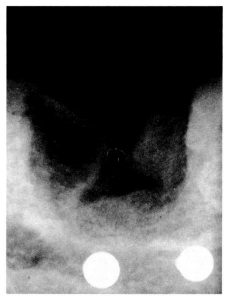

3-32

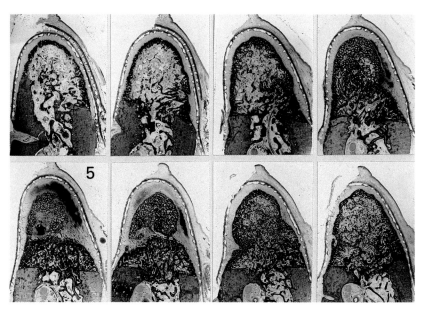

3-33

the membrane-bound space. Sequential radiographs demonstrate how bone grows from the bottom and from the mesial and distal walls into the middle portion of the defect. The membrane itself initially is not accepted as a base for bone deposition and, in most of the cases, stays separated from the bone surface by an interposed connective tissue layer. In serial coronal sections, the fine structure of the regenerate reveals remarkable structural modifications. Close to the mesial wall, bone is attached to the existing cortical layer and confines a uniform marrow space (Fig 3-33, upper left). Toward the middle portion, this space is sealed by a coherent layer of spongiosa, which is already contiguous with the corresponding part in the distal portion. The third center of bone formation is in the bottom of the defect (Fig 3-34). Similar to the controls, a bony seal has formed across the opening of the marrow cavity. This dome-shaped seal has already fused with the distal portion of the regenerate but not yet with its mesial counterpart, where a thin layer of fibrous tissue separates the two components.

Formation of the Primary Spongework

The microscopic aspect of bone formation in the membrane-protected area exhibits a remarkable similarity to bone development and growth (Fig 3-35). The organization of the hematoma by granulation tissue follows the basic pattern of wound healing. The invading vascular sprouts are accompanied by cells originating from the bone marrow around the defect. Bone marrow stroma cells belong to the category of determined osteoprecursor cells (page 68) and, when activated, become the source of osteoblast precursors. During invasion and organization of the hematoma, these inconspicuous cells can only be characterized by their perivascular location and the result of their activation, which is ultimately bone formation. The majority of the vessels resemble sinusoidal capillaries or thin-walled veins. They are integrated into a finely meshed net by frequent anastomoses. From the cut cortical and trabecular surfaces, woven bone sprouts out, mostly in the shape of thin, bifurcating plates (Fig 3-36). These trabeculae advance between the blood vessels, surround them, and then fuse again, thereby confining an intertrabecular space. Initially, the trabeculae consist of osteoid only. Then mineralization starts in the center and separates the future osteoid seams. The osteoid surface is covered by an uninterrupted layer of osteoblasts that extends, together with the osteoid seams, into the deeper intertrabecular meshes of the bony regenerate.

From its overall architecture, one is tempted to designate the newly formed bone as a primary spongiosa. This term, however, refers originally to cancellous bone that originates from endochondral ossification in secondary epiphyseal ossification centers or in growth plates. The primary spongiosa always encloses remnants of calcified cartilage and is also referred to as the "chondro-osseous complex." The bony scaffold formed beneath the mem-

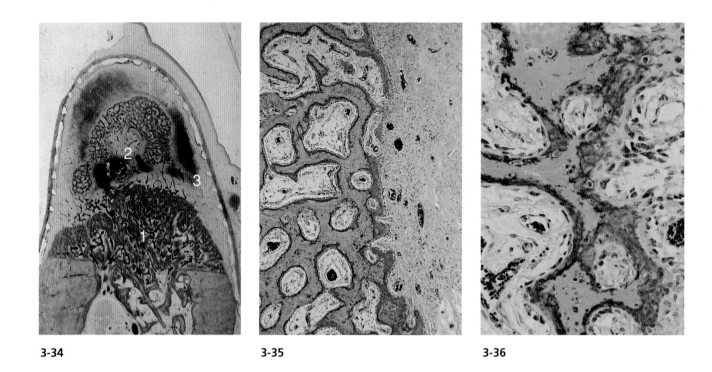

3-34   3-35   3-36

Fig 3-34 Section no. 5 from Fig 3-33 shows (1) the bony cover of the bottom marrow space and (2) a tangential section through the top of the bony hill originating from the mesial wall of the defect, as well as the associated hematoma (3). Magnification × 4

Fig 3-35 Organization of the hematoma and woven bone formation. Blood vessels and bone-forming cells invade the former hematoma *(at right)* and construct a scaffold of woven bone. Goldner's trichrome stain; Magnification × 20.

Fig 3-36 In the advancing ossification front, blood vessels and outgrowing trabeculae are tightly interconnected. (Goldner's trichrome stains osteoid seams red, mineralized bone green.) Magnification × 90.

brane, however, has no cartilaginous precursor and is, in fact, a primarily or directly formed bone, resulting from a sort of intramembranous ossification. In view of its further differentiation and elaboration, herein it will be referred to as "primary scaffold" or, as in earlier decades, "primary spongework."[73]

The primary spongework also diverges from regular spongiosa in other respects. Structurally, it is perfectly isotropic, ie, the trabeculae have no preferential orientation (Fig 3-37). Its dimensions are also different: Porosity is slightly below 50% (adult spongiosa 70% to 80%), the mean diameter of the trabeculae is about 60 μm (adult about 200 μm), and the "pore size" (mean width of intertrabecular spaces) ranges from 100 to 200 μm (adult about 500 μm).

The contents of the intertrabecular spaces are noteworthy too. The main constituents are the large, thin-walled blood vessels that have been incorporated during the formation of the primary spongework. The bony scaffold and the vascular plexus are perfectly interdigitated. It becomes difficult to judge which component has taken the lead in determining the architecture of this framework. In an advancing ossification front, the blood vessels always precede the osteoblasts. In addition, osteoblasts derive from perivascular cells and function only in the vicinity of capillaries. It is plausible that the vascular network plays a certain role for the orientation of the bony elements in the primary spongework, although bone itself may possess an inherent growth pattern (cf also the classical dispute of this topic, as summarized by Murray,[73] or Krompecher's hypothesis of a "primary angiogenic ossification"[74]).

Further Development of the Primary Spongework

Originally, the primary spongework consists exclusively of woven bone. In its further development it serves as a template for the development of compact bone as well as for a transformation into a regular spongiosa (Figs 3-38 and 3-39).

Formation of a **cortical layer** and development of a regular spongiosa and marrow space are the major events in the third and fourth months after surgery (Figs 3-40 and 3-41). The formation of a peripheral cortical bone layer starts in the vicinity of the mesial and distal walls of the defect as a continuation of the original cortex. From there it advances toward the middle portion.

The surface of the trabeculae in the primary spongework is lined by a coherent layer of active osteoblasts (Fig 3-42a). Continuous bone deposition increases the diameter of the trabeculae and narrows the intertrabecular spaces (Figs 3-42b and c). The structure of the newly formed bone changes gradually from woven to lamellar bone, parallel-fibered bone being an intermediate stage of this maturation (page 59). The endpoint of this process is reached when the former intertrabecular spaces attain the size of regular cortical canals and, together with the surrounding concentric lamellae, constitute primary osteons (Fig 3-42d).

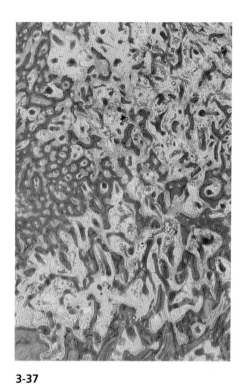

3-37

Fig 3-37 Structure of the primary spongework after 2 months. Numerous vessels have grown in from the underlying marrow space (the veins are tightly filled with blood and appear yellow-brown). The trabeculae construct an isotropic scaffold. Ground section, toluidine blue surface stain; magnification × 12.

Fig 3-38 Radiograph of membrane-covered defect after 4 months. (Reprinted with permission from Schenk et al.[71])

Fig 3-39 Selected buccolingual sections, cut at intervals of 1.5 mm, arranged in a distal-mesial sequence. Section nos. 1 and 8 pass through the distal and the mesial wall of the defect. Magnification × 1.2. (Reprinted with permission from Schenk et al.[71])

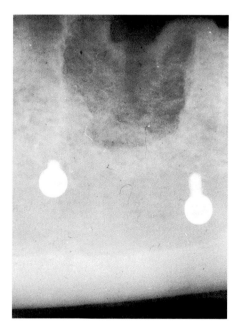

3-38

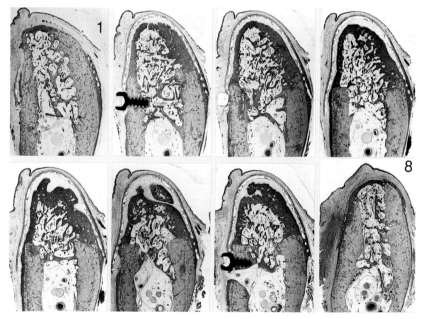

3-39

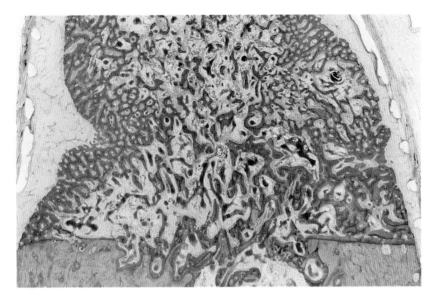

3-40

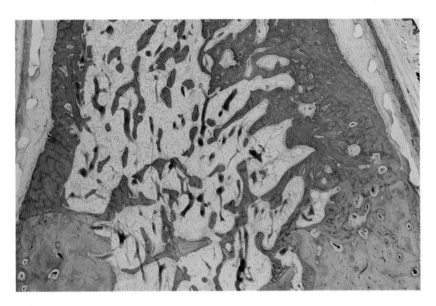

3-41

Fig 3-40 Transformation of the primary spongework into cortical bone and cancellous bone. After 2 months, the peripheral spongiosa is somewhat denser than in the center. Magnification × 9.

Fig 3-41 Cortical bone and secondary spongiosa after 4 months. A compact bone layer in the periphery confines a cancellous bone in the center with well-defined trabeculae and regular bone marrow. Toluidine blue surface stain; magnification × 9.

Formation and maturation of cortical bone.
Figs 3-42a to d

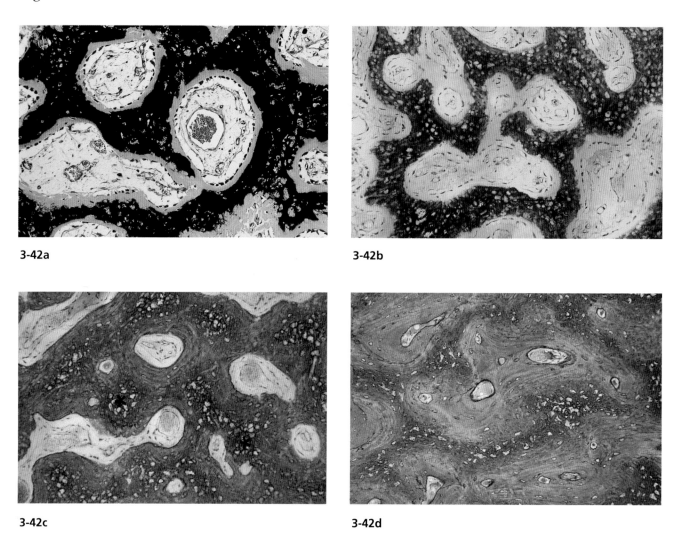

3-42a

3-42b

3-42c

3-42d

Fig 3-42a Newly formed woven bone, covered by a continuous layer of osteoblasts, surrounds well-vascularized intertrabecular spaces. Microtome section, von Kossa-McNeal stain; magnification × 90. (Reprinted with permission from Schenk et al.[71])

Fig 3-42b Newly formed woven bone, same as in Fig 3-42a. Ground section, toluidine blue surface stain; magnification × 90. (Reprinted with permission from Schenk et al.[71])

Fig 3-42c Reinforcement of woven bone *(asterisks)* by parallel-fibered bone, 2 months after surgery. Surface staining with toluidine blue; magnification × 90. (Reprinted with permission from Schenk et al.[71])

Fig 3-42d Transformation into primary osteons by continuous filling of the intertrabecular spaces, 4 months after surgery. Woven bone is still clearly recognizable. Surface staining with toluidine blue; magnification × 90. (Reprinted with permission from Schenk et al.[71])

Formation of secondary spongiosa. *Figs 3-43a and b*

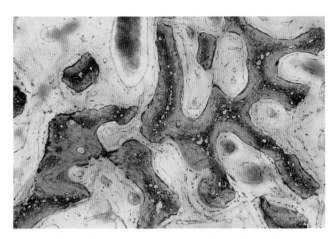

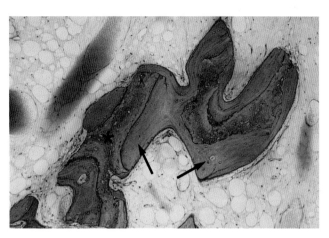

Fig 3-43a After 2 months, the trabeculae of the primary spongework consist of woven bone, reinforced by a layer of parallel-fibered bone. Toluidine blue surface stain; magnification × 75.

Fig 3-43b After 4 months, remodeling results in trabeculae that are composed of remnants of the original scaffold *(asterisk)*, covered by packets of lamellar bone *(arrows)*. Magnification × 75.

Formation of a **secondary spongiosa** starts in the center of the coronal sections, where the marrow space expands by resorption of the primary spongework (Fig 3-43a). The spared trabeculae undergo profound remodeling, and the remnants of woven and parallel-fibered bone are gradually replaced by packets of lamellar bone (Fig 3-43b, see also page 65). This process too starts mesially and distally and proceeds into the middle portion. The resulting cancellous bone is contiguous with pre-existing trabeculae in the walls of the defect.

Cortical Bone Remodeling
During the fourth month, the cortical bone enters its last phase of differentiation, ie, haversian remodeling. Activation of BMUs (page 65) leads to the formation of resorption canals, which subsequently are filled by concentric lamellae (Figs 3-44a and b). The resulting secondary osteons are clearly differentiated from primary osteons by the surrounding cement lines of the reversal type (Fig 3-44c). The remodeling process also starts in the most mature part of the regenerate, ie, close to the margins of the defect, and gradually progresses into the middle portion and from the bottom toward the roof of the reconstructed cortical wall.

Modeling of the Bony Regenerate
At the end of the fourth month, growth and modeling of the bone within the membrane-confined volume continues, especially in the middle portion. With the formation of a cortical bone layer, the periosteal and endosteal envelopes have also been restored.

Cortical bone remodeling. *Figs 3-44a to c*

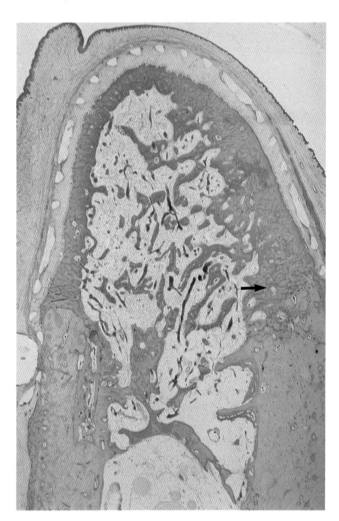

3-44a

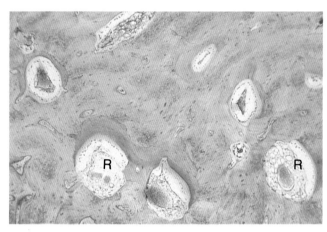

3-44b

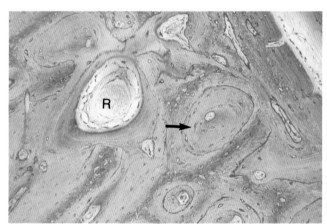

3-44c

Fig 3-44a At 4 months, haversian remodeling starts within the compact cortical layer, preferentially in the vicinity of the original cortex *(arrow)*. Magnification × 6.

Fig 3-44b Initially formed resorption canals (R) are refilled with mature lamellar bone. Magnification × 45.

Fig 3-44c Higher magnification shows a resorption canal with beginning bone deposition (R), and a completed secondary osteon, confined by a cement line *(arrow)*. Magnification ×90.

Modeling of the cortical bone. *Figs 3-45a and b*

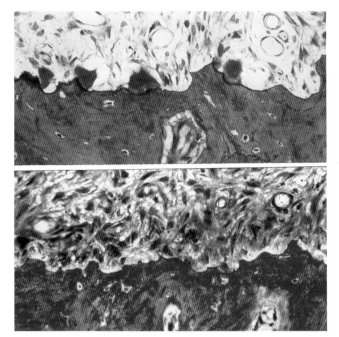

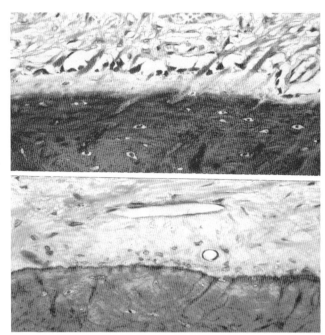

Fig 3-45a *Top:* Active, ongoing resorption is indicated by the presence of osteoclasts. *Bottom:* Howship's lacunae, or an eroded surface, persist after osteoclastic resorption, until they are covered by newly formed bone. Magnification × 320.

Fig 3-45b *Top:* Osteoblasts and osteoid seams indicate bone apposition. *Bottom:* Resting or quiescent surfaces are lined by a regular periosteum. Magnification × 320.

They resume their modeling activities by means of shape-deforming resorption and formation along the outer and inner cortical surfaces (Figs 3-45a and b). As long as modeling is going on, the bone surface is locally lined by osteoblasts and osteoid seams, or is covered by osteoclasts or Howship's lacunae, as a sign of ongoing or past resorption. In quiescent sites the bone surface is smooth, and collagen is incorporated as Sharpey's fibers in the mineralized bone matrix. In all of the remodeling sites, the number of blood vessels increases. As a result, the surface of the cortex becomes more clearly defined and the intertrabecular spaces better interconnected. Thereby, the gradient of maturation is maintained; the middle portion always lags somewhat behind in view of overall height, bone density, and organization.

Soft Tissue Compartments

Installation of barrier membranes promotes bone repair mainly by protection of the defect against invasion by competing, less differentiated and rapidly proliferating cells. In our experiments, the membrane covers a surgically produced defect in the alveolar process in the mandible, in a site where the teeth had previously been removed. The membrane is closely adapted to the bony margins surrounding the defect and, thanks to its stiffness, forms a rather stable wall of a tunnel with a volume of about 1 cm³.

The bone regeneration within the membrane-protected space has already been described. This section deals with the soft tissue differentiation inside and outside the membrane barrier and along the membrane-tissue interface (Fig 3-46a).

Histologically, the connective tissue in the outer compartment appears to be characteristic of a normal keratinized gingiva and oral mucosa (Fig 3-46b). The connective tissue in the lamina propria contains slender collagen fibers. Toward the membrane, the density and the diameter of the fibers increases, and coarse bundles of collagen establish contact with the surface of the e-PTFE membrane. Throughout the inner compartment, loose connective tissue with delicate collagen fibrils predominates (Fig 3-46c). This tissue is derived from bone marrow. It is well vascularized and the number of vessels increases toward the bone surface. Among the cellular elements, the fixed cells clearly outweigh the mobile elements. Macrophages, lymphocytes, or granulocytes are extremely rare, even in contact with the inner surface of the membrane. This again provides proof of the excellent tissue compatibility of the e-PTFE membrane.

The width of the inner connective tissue compartment, ie, the distance between the inner surface of the membrane and the periosteal envelope, varies considerably. As a rule, it is small in the mesial and distal portions and gets larger in the middle portion. As expected, it is thicker at 2 months and diminishes at 3 and 4 months. This is partially due to continued periosteal bone apposition. However, the stiffness of the membrane might also play a role: In the relatively large defects, the reinforced membranes are less subject to deformation and almost fully preserve the space created during surgery. Some of the nonreinforced membranes, on the other hand, have been slightly deformed and, thereby, the space underneath the membrane locally collapsed.

The design of the e-PTFE membranes used in our experiments provides a certain porosity, with communicating interstices approximately 50 μm in diameter (see Chapter 4). This pore size allows invasion by cells and small vessels, and it seems appropriate to define a third, "intra-GORE-TEX-membranous" compartment, since practically all porous parts are populated with living cells (Figs 3-47 and 3-48). Most of these are fibroblasts and are accompanied by thin collagen fibers and small capillaries. Of special interest are sections where the membrane has come into close contact with bone. This is the case toward the bottom of the defect, where the membrane was pressed on the original periosteum by the miniscrews, or in sites where outgrowing bone has established direct contact with the inner surface of the membrane (Fig 3-49). In such sites, bone has grown into the pores and interstices. Bone is directly deposited on the pore walls, fills the pores almost completely, and penetrates through the membrane (Fig 3-50). The bony filling is not restricted to the immediate contact area with

Soft tissue compartments.   *Figs 3-46a to c*

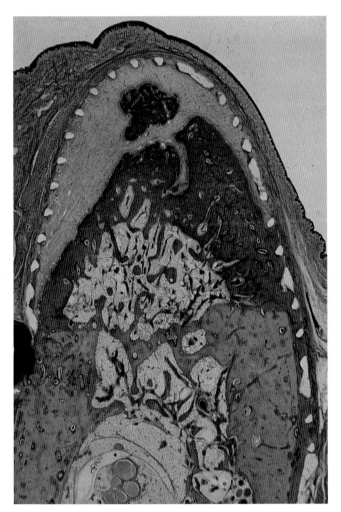

3-46a

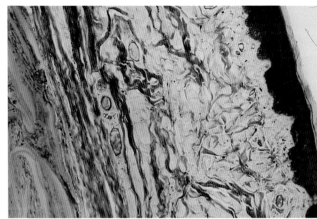

3-46b

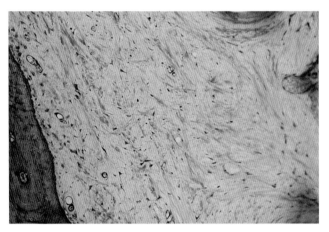

3-46c

Fig 3-46a   The (reinforced) membrane separates an outer, gingival compartment from the compartment that is mainly accessible from the marrow space. Magnification × 6.

Fig 3-46b   The outer compartment is lined by the gingival epithelium. The lamina propria is characterized by fibrous connective tissue with collagen fibrils of increasing diameter toward the membrane. Magnification × 90.

Fig 3-46c   In the inner compartment the well-vascularized loose connective tissue is derived from the bone marrow. Along the bone surface it forms the periosteal envelope. Magnification × 90.

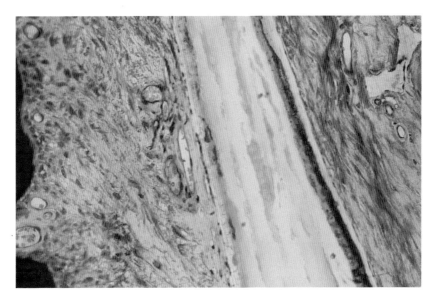

3-47

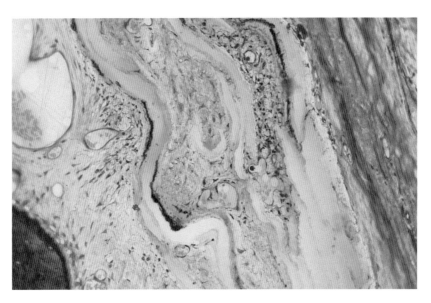

3-48

Fig 3-47 Nonreinforced membrane has a dense central and a porous peripheral part. Its surface is in direct contact with the adjacent fibrous tissue; there are no signs of any foreign-body reaction. Magnification × 200.

Fig 3-48 The porous part of the nonreinforced membrane allows ingrowth of vessels and cells into the membrane interstices. Magnification × 200.

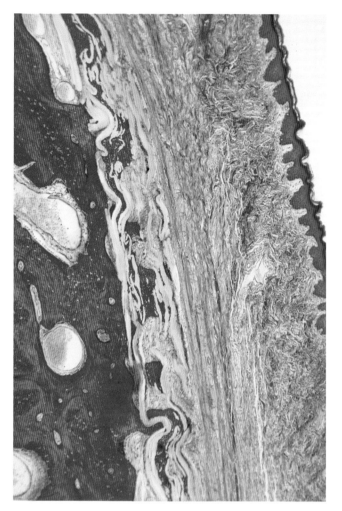

3-49

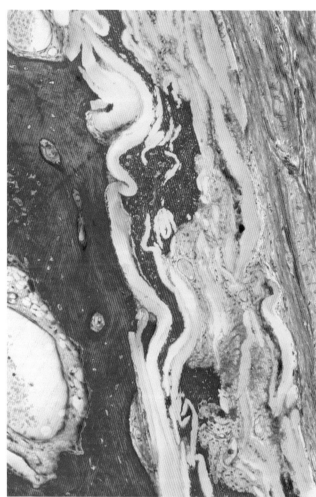

3-50

Fig 3-49 Newly formed bone makes contact with the inner surface of the membrane, and bone formation starts filling the interstices of the membrane pores. Ground section, toluidine blue and basic fuchsin stain; magnification × 50.

Fig 3-50 Higher magnification of Fig 3-49 shows direct bony ongrowth on the inner surface of the membrane, and bony ingrowth into its pores; magnification × 180.

the underlying bone, but spreads out on both sides over a remarkable distance. This "intramembranous" ossification again shows that the membrane consists of a perfectly bioinert material and may have osteoconductive properties. In addition, the osteogenic potential of the invading cells suggests that they ultimately derive from bone marrow stroma cells and that marrow-borne cells indeed represent the vast majority of the cell population in the former defect area, including the interstices of the membrane.

Summary

Among the highly organized tissues, bone has the unique potential to rebuild its original structure after a defect or fracture. The pattern of bone healing closely resembles development and growth. In unstable conditions, indirect or secondary healing via intermediate fibrocartilage formation followed by endochondral ossification predominates. In stable conditions, bone is formed directly or primarily, provided that two essential conditions are fulfilled: ample blood supply and a solid base for bone depositions. The solid base is furnished by the surface of the fragment ends or by the bony margins of a defect.

Repair of bone defects closely resembles appositional growth. In the initial, rapid phase, a template of woven bone is constructed and is gradually reinforced by lamellar bone. In accordance with the local environment, this primary spongework is then transformed into compact cortical or trabecular bone. In the second phase, the regenerate undergoes profound remodeling and substitution by remodeling units (BMUs). In cortical bone, the remodeling units construct secondary osteons. In cancellous bone, the resulting bone structural units (BSUs) form "packets."

While healing of bone defects has size limits, which are in the range of a couple of millimeters, there are means to promote bone regeneration:

- **Osteoconduction** facilitates bridging of larger defects by offering a solid scaffold for bone deposition and later substitution.

- **Distraction osteogenesis** yields impressive results by canalizing bony callus formation into longitudinal compartments, confined by continuously stretched collagen fiber bundles.

- **Guided bone regeneration** is the most recent achievement, based on a hitherto neglected principle: the protection of bone regeneration against overgrowth by rapidly proliferating non-osteogenic tissues. It is successfully applied for alveolar ridge augmentation, whereby barrier membranes create a secluded space for invasion of blood vessels and osteoprogenitor cells. The membrane protects the invading elements against competing fibroblasts originating in the gingival mucosa.

References

1. Palumbo C, Palazzini S, Zaffe D, Marotti D. Osteocyte differentiation in the tibia of newborn rabbits: An ultrastructural study of the formation of cytoplasmic processes. Acta Anat 1990;137:350.

2. Frost HM. Bone Remodeling Dynamics. Springfield, IL: Charles C Thomas, 1963.

3. Frost HM. Bone Dynamics in Osteoporosis and Osteomalacia. Springfield, IL: Charles C Thomas, 1966.

4. Frost HM. Micropetrosis. J Bone Joint Surg 1960;42A:144.

5. Parfitt AM. Quantum concept of bone remodeling and turnover: Implications for the pathogenesis of osteoporosis. Calcif Tissue Int 1979;28:1.

6. Parfitt AM. The coupling of bone formation to bone resorption: A critical analysis of the concept and of its relevance to the pathogenesis of osteoporosis. Metab Bone Dis Relat Res 1982;4:1.

7. Price P, Parthemore J, Deftos J. New biochemical marker for bone metabolism. J Clin Invest 1980;66:878.

8. Oldberg A, Franzen A, Heinegard D. Cloning and sequence analysis of rat bone sialoprotein (osteopontin). cDNA reveals an Arg-Gly-Asp cell-binding sequence. Proc Natl Acad Sci USA 1986;83:8819.

9. Reinholt FP, Hultenby K, Oldberg A, Heinegård D. Osteopontin—A possible anchor of osteoclasts to bone. Proc Natl Acad Sci USA 1990;87:4473–4475.

10. Termine J, Kleinman H, Whitson W, Conn K, McGarvey M, Martin G. Osteonectin, a bone-specific protein linking mineral to collagen. Cell 1981;26:99.

11. Boskey AL. Non-collagenous matrix proteins and their role in mineralisation. Bone Miner 1989;6:111 (RD 44).

12. Anderson HC. Mechanism of mineral formation in bone. Lab Invest 1989;60:320.

13. Kahn AJ, Fallon MD, Teitelbaum SL. Structure-function relationships in bone: An examination of events at the cellular level. In: Peck WA (ed). Bone and Mineral Research, Annual 2. Amsterdam: Elsevier, 1983:125–174.

14. Glimcher MJ. Molecular biology of mineralized tissues with particular reference to bone. Rev Mod Phys 1959;31:359.

15. Glimcher MJ. Compositions, structure and organization of bone and other mineralized tissues and the mechanism of calcification. In: Aurbach GB (ed). Handbook of Physiology-Endocrinology VII. Baltimore: Williams and Wilkins, 1976:25–166.

16. Glimcher MJ. The possible role of collagen fibrils and collagen-phosphoprotein complexes in the calcification of bone in vitro and in vivo. Biomaterials 1989;11:7.

17. Jones SJ, Boyde A. Scanning electron microscopy of bone cells in cultures. In: Copp DH, Talmage RV (eds). Endocrinology of Calcium Metabolism. Amsterdam: Excerpta Medica, 1978:97–104.

18. Ham AW. Some histophysiological problems peculiar to calcified tissues. J Bone Joint Surg 1952;34A:701.

19. Frost HM. Measurements of osteocytes per unit volume and volume components of osteocytes and canaliculae in man. Henry Ford Hosp Med Bull 1960;8:208.

20. Chappard D, Alexandre C, Riffat G. Histochemical identification of osteoclasts. Review of current methods and reappraisal of a simple procedure for routine diagnosis on undecalcified human iliac bone biopsies. Basic Appl Histochem 1983;27:75.

21. Minkin C. Bone acid phosphatase: Tartrate-resistant acid phosphatase as a marker of osteoclast function. Calcif Tissue Int 1982;34:285.

22. Kölliker A. Die normale Resorption des Knochengewebes und ihre Bedeutung für die Entstehung der typischen Knochenformen. Leipzig, Germany: FCW Vogel, 1873.

23. Holtrop ME, King GJ. The ultrastructure of the osteoclast and its functional implications. Clin Orthop 1977;123:177.

24. Vaes G. Cellular biology and biochemical mechanism of bone resorption. Clin Orthop 1988;231:239.

25. Marks SC, Popoff SN. Ultrastructural biology and pathology of the osteoclasts. In: Bonucci E, Motta PM (eds). Ultrastructure of Skeletal Tissues. Dordrecht, Netherlands: Kluwer, 1990:239–252.

26. Takahashi N, Akatsu T, Udagawa N, Sasaki T, Yamaguchi A, Moseley JM, et al. Osteoblastic cells are involved in osteoclast formation. Endocrinology 1988; 123:2600.

27. Kurihara N, Cheni C, Miller M, Civin C, Roodman GD. Identification of committed mononuclear precursors for osteoclast-like cells formed in long term human marrow cultures. Endocrinology 1990;126:2733.

28. Martin TJ, Ng KW, Suda T. Bone cell physiology. Endocrinol Metab Clin North Am 1989;18:833.

29. Jaworski ZF, Duck B, Sekaly G. Kinetics of osteoclasts and their nuclei in evolving secondary Haversian systems. J Anat 1981;133:397.

30. Schenk RK. Basic histomorphology and physiology of skeletal growth. In: Weber BG, Brunner C, Freuler F (eds). Treatment of Fractures in Children and Adolescents. Berlin: Springer, 1980:3–19.

31. Schenk RK. Biology of fracture repair. In: Browner BD, Jupiter JB, Levine AM, Traften PG (eds). Skeletal Trauma. Philadelphia: Saunders, 1992:31–75.

32. Hunziker EB, Schenk RK, Cruz-Orive LM. Quantitation of chondrocyte performance in growth-plate cartilage during longitudinal bone growth. J Bone Joint Surg 1987;69-A:162.

33. Hunziker EB, Schenk RK. Physiological mechanisms adopted by chondrocytes in regulating longitudinal bone growth in rats. J Physiol 1989;414:55.

34. Enlow DH. Functions of the Haversian system. Am J Anat 1962;110:269.

35. Currey JD. Some effects of aging in human Haversian systems. J Anat 1964;98:69.

36. Jaworski ZF, Lok E. The rate of osteoclastic bone erosion in Haversian remodeling sites of adult dog's rib. Calcif Tissue Res 1972;10:103.

37. Schenk R, Willenegger H. Morphological findings in primary fracture healing. In: Krompecher S, Kerner E (eds). Callus Formation: Symposium on the Biology of Fracture Healing. Symp Biologica Hungarica 1967;7:75–86.

38. Schenk RK. Cytodynamics and histodynamics of primary bone repair. In: Lane JM (ed). Fracture Healing. Edinburgh: Churchill Livingstone, 1987:23–32.

39. Brookes M, Harrison RG. The vascularization of the rabbit femur and tibiofibula. J Anat 1957;91:61.

40. Wolff J. Das Gesetz der Transformation der Knochen. Berlin: Hirschwalk, 1892.

41. Drivdahl RH, Howard GA, Baylink DJ. Extracts of bone contain a potent regulator of bone formation. Biochem Biophys Acta 1982;724:26.

42. Mundy GR. Inflammatory mediators and the destruction of bone. J Periodont Res 1991;26:213.

43. Frost HM. Dynamics of bone remodelling. In: Frost HM (ed). Bone Biodynamics. Boston: Little, Brown, 1964:315–333.

44. Lacroix P. Organizers and growth of bone. J Bone Joint Surg 1947;29:292.

45. Urist MR, McLean FC. Osteogenetic potency and new-bone formation by induction in transplants to the anterior chamber of the eye. J Bone Joint Surg 1952;34-A:443.

46. Urist MR, Silbermann BF, Buring K, Dubuc FL, Rosenberg JM. The bone inducting principle. Clin Orthop Rel Res 1967;53:243.

47. Wozney JM. Role of the BMP family of proteins in osteoinduction. In: American Society for Bone and Mineral Research, Workshop C: Calcified Tissue Matrix: Composition and Regulation. 1990;17–27.

48. Friedenstein A. Determined and inducible osteogenic precursor cells. In: Elliott K, Fitzsimmons D (eds). Hard Tissue Growth, Repair, and Remineralization; Ciba Foundation Symposium 1973;11:169–185.

49. Friedenstein AJ. Precursor cells of mechanocytes. Int Rev Cytol 1976;47:327.

50. Reddi AH. Cell biology and biochemistry of endochondral bone development. Coll Res 1981;1:209.

51. Johner R. Zur Knochenheilung in Abhängigkeit von der Defektgrösse. Helv Chir Acta 1972;39:409.

52. Schenk R, Willenegger H. Zur Histologie der primären Knochenheilung. Modifikationen und Grenzen der Spaltheilung in Abhängigkeit von der Defektgrösse. Unfallheilkunde 1977;80:155.

53. Harris WJ, White RE, McCarthy JC, Walker PS, Weinberg EH. Bony ingrowth fixation of the acetabular component in canine hip joint arthroplasty. Clin Orthop 1983;176:7.

54. Schenk RK, Müller J, Willenegger H. Experimentell-histologischer Beitrag zur Entstehung und Behandlung von Pseudarthrosen. H Unfallheilk 1968;94:15.

55. Eggli PS, Müller W, Schenk RK. Porous hydroxyapatite and tricalcium phosphate cylinders with two different pore size ranges implanted in the cancellous bone of rabbits. A comparative histomorphometric and histologic study of bony ingrowth and implant substitution. Clin Orthop Rel Res 1988;232:127.

56. Ilizarov GA. The tension-stress effect on the genesis and growth of tissues, part I. The influence of stability on fixation and soft-tissue preservation. Clin Orthop 1989;238:249

57. Ilizarov GA. The tension-stress effect on the genesis and growth of tissues, part II. The influence of rate and frequency of distraction. Clin Orthop 1989;239:263.

58. Paterson D. Leg-lengthening procedures: A historical review. Clin Orthop 1990;250:27.

59. Aronson J, Harrison BH, Steward CL, Harp JH. The histology of distraction osteogenesis using different external fixators. Clin Orthop 1989;241:106.

60. Delloye C, Delefortrie G, Coutelier L, Vincent A. Bone regenerate formation in cortical bone during distraction lengthening: An experimental study. Clin Orthop 1989;250:34.

61. Shearer JR, Roach HI, Parsons SW. Histology of a lengthened human tibia. J Bone Joint Surg 1992;74-B:39.

62. Hurley LA, Stinchfield FE, Bassett CAL, Lyon WH. The role of soft tissues in osteogenesis. J Bone Joint Surg 1959;41-A:1243.

63. Boyne PJ. Regeneration of alveolar bone beneath cellulose acetate filter implants. J Dent Res 1964;26:569.

64. Nyman S, Lindhe J, Karring T. Reattachment-new attachment. In: Lindhe J (ed). Textbook of Clinical Periodontology, ed 2. Copenhagen: Munksgard, 1989:450–476.

65. Dahlin C, Linde A, Gottlow J, Nyman S. Healing of bone defects by guided tissue regeneration. Plast Reconstr Surg 1988;81:672.

66. Dahlin C, Gottlow J, Linde A, Nyman S. Healing of maxillary and mandibular bone defects using a membrane technique. Scand J Plast Reconstr Hand Surg 1990;24:13.

67. Seibert J, Nyman S. Localized ridge augmentation in dogs: A pilot study using membranes and hydroxylapatite. J Periodontol 1990;61:157.

68. Becker W, Becker B, Handlesman M, Celletti R, Ochsenbein C, Hardwick R, et al. Bone formation at dehisced dental implant sites treated with implant augmentation material: A pilot study in dogs. Int J Periodont Rest Dent 1990;10:93.

69. Nyman S, Lang NP, Buser D, Brägger U. Bone regeneration adjacent to titanium dental implants using guided tissue regeneration. Int J Oral Maxillofac Implants 1990;5:9.

70. Buser D, Dula K, Belser U, Hirt HP, Berthold H. Localized Ridge Augmentation Using Guided Bone Regeneration. I. Surgical Procedure in the Maxilla. Int J Periodont Rest Dent 1993;13:29.

71. Schenk RK, Buser D, Hardwick WR, Dahlin C. Healing pattern of bone regeneration in membrane-protected defects. A histologic study in the canine mandible. Int J Oral Maxillofac Implants 1994;9:13–29.

72. Schenk RK, Olah AJ, Herrmann W. Preparation of calcified tissues for light microscopy. In: Dickson GR (ed). Methods of Calcified Tissue Preparation. Amsterdam: Elsevier, 1984:1–56.

73. Murray PDF. Bones. A Study of the Development and Structure of the Vertebrate Skeleton. Cambridge: University Press, 1936.

74. Krompecher ST. Die Knochenbildung. Jena, Germany: Gustav Fischer, 1937.

CHAPTER FOUR

Membrane Design Criteria for Guided Bone Regeneration of the Alveolar Ridge

Ross Hardwick
Todd V. Scantlebury
Raquel Sanchez
Nancy Whitley
Jeanne Ambruster

The recent acceptance of membrane-assisted regeneration of oral osseous tissue has introduced reconstructive dentistry to new therapeutic procedures and biomaterials. As this therapy gains wider practice, clinicians will be exposed to an increasing number of membrane materials used, or proposed for use, in guided bone regeneration (GBR). To select the material(s) best suited to a specific clinical application and to achieve the optimal therapeutic results for patients, it is necessary to understand the functional requirements demanded of membrane materials used in GBR procedures.

Because the focus of this book is on GBR in implant dentistry, discussion in this chapter is limited to the functional requirements of membrane materials intended for use in regeneration of the alveolar ridge. The GBR procedures performed in the alveolar process pose specific challenges that must be addressed in membrane design if the membrane is to function at the optimal level in clinical use.

The guiding principle of functional anatomy is encompassed in the phrase "form follows function." To perform a particular function, an anatomic structure must possess certain specific characteristics. For example, the primary functions of the human hand are grasping and the capability for precise manipulation of objects. The anatomic structures and physiologic activities that permit these functions are specific to the functions and are extremely complex.

Medical devices must also have specific attributes or characteristics that allow performance of the intended function. For example, a prosthetic vascular graft must have very different characteristics than those of a prosthetic anterior cruciate ligament.

For a medical device to perform its primary function(s) at the optimal level, it is first necessary to identify the critical requirements for function. These requirements are based on biologic, mechanical, and clinical use factors, and optimal device design will take each of these factors into account. Once the critical requirements have been identified, the desired structural and chemical characteristics that will allow the device to meet these requirements must be incorporated into the design.

As described in detail in Chapters 2 and 3, use of an occlusive or semi-occlusive membrane to provide a protected, blood clot–filled space adjacent to a bony surface will result in fill of that space by bone tissue.[1-4] The prevailing rationale for this phenomenon is that the membrane, by acting as a physical barrier, prevents ingrowth of fibrous connective tissue (scar) into the space. As a result, osteogenic cells originating from the bone, and supported by adequate vascularity, are allowed to repopulate the space.

If the only requirement of a membrane material used for GBR procedures were to provide a barrier to the proliferation of fibrous connective tissue, any suitably biocompatible material in the form of a cell-occlusive film could be utilized in clinical practice. However, a membrane that is utilized for alveolar ridge GBR must meet a number of requirements in addition to acting as a passive physical barrier.

This chapter discusses each of these requirements in detail and identifies some of the biomaterial design solutions that may be used to meet these requirements and optimize membrane function. Because much of what is known about the functional requirements of membranes for alveolar ridge GBR has been learned in the development of membrane materials for periodontal applications, some examples from periodontal research are used. However, because of application-specific requirements, an alveolar ridge GBR membrane will not look or function exactly like a membrane designed for periodontal applications.

Membrane Requirements for GBR of the Alveolar Ridge

1. The membrane must be constructed of acceptably **biocompatible** material(s). The interaction between the material and tissue should not adversely affect the surrounding tissue, the intended healing result, or the overall safety of the patient.

2. The membrane should exhibit suitable **occlusive** properties to prevent fibrous connective tissue (scar) invasion of the space adjacent to the bone and provide some degree of protection from bacterial invasion should the membrane become exposed to the oral environment.

3. The membrane must be able to provide a suitable space into which osseous regeneration can occur. **Spacemaking** provides necessary volume with specific geometry for functional reconstruction.

4. The membrane should be capable of integrating with or attaching to the surrounding tissue. **Tissue integration** helps to stabilize the healing wound, helps to create a "seal" between the bone and the material and prevent fibrous connective tissue leakage into the defect, and retards the migration of epithelium around the material should it become exposed.

5. The membrane must be **clinically manageable.**

Biocompatibility

Biocompatibility is a fundamental requirement for acceptable function of any implantable medical device. Although this requirement is often taken for granted, tissue-biomaterial interactions involve many application-specific factors that are governed by complex and, in many ways, poorly understood mechanisms.

Williams[5] defines biocompatibility as, ". . . the state of affairs when a biomaterial exists within a physiological environment, without the material adversely and significantly affecting the body, or the environment of the body adversely and significantly affecting the material." This definition, however useful, must be interpreted with respect to the biomaterial used, the intended function(s) of the device, and the environment into which the material is placed and maintained. For example, degradable materials are clearly affected by the environment of the body; however, safe degradation is one of the primary intended functions of this class of biomaterials.

Understanding the biocompatibility characteristics of a device that will be implanted in a patient is crucial, because biomaterial-host interactions play a critical role in the device's capacity to perform its intended function(s). Devices such as bone-anchored (osseointegrated) dental implants and vascular prostheses depend on specific and predictable biomaterial-host interaction for long-term function. At the very least, biomaterial-host interactions should not interfere with the ability of a given device to perform its intended function, and should not present significant safety concerns for the patient.

Biocompatibility is a relative term. All implanted materials, regardless of composition, interact with the host to some degree. Biomaterials of dissimilar chemical composition, or even biomaterials with the same base chemical composition but with different microstructures and macrostructures, may exhibit different levels of cellular or systemic response.[6] Figure 4-1 shows three well-known biomaterials implanted into the same tissue bed and exhibiting different levels of tissue response.

Biocompatibility is, therefore, a fundamental concern in device design and must be evaluated with respect to the requirements of the application. In this context the following discussion focuses on the biocompatibility characteristics that allow GBR membranes to function optimally in alveolar ridge regeneration.

Biocompatibility and Patient Safety

Patient safety is the foremost concern in the selection of a biomaterial as a potential GBR membrane. Extensive testing is required to ensure the safety of a biomaterial, and long-term clinical experience may be helpful in selecting an appropriate material or device. Standards for biocompatibility testing that reflect current thought regarding safety standards have been established. For example, the Tripartite Biocompatibility Guidance for Medical Devices[7] represents biocompatibility testing standards set by the United States, Canada, and the United Kingdom. Appropriate biocompatibility testing is dependent on the type of material and clinical application, and clinicians should be aware of the scope and applicability of tests performed on a device that is made available for clinical use.

Assuming the use of appropriate base components, acceptable purity, and appropriate structure, inert materials (those that do not degrade chemically in physiologic conditions) generally present a less complex safety situation than degradable materials. As long as an inert biomaterial remains intact (not broken up or particulated by mechanical forces), the material will not release potentially harmful by-products into the host. Chemically inert materials may contain contaminants, but these may be bound up in the material structure and only those located at the surface are available for interaction with the host. However, it is important to

know whether leaching of impurities will occur and what effect these substances may have on the host. Currently, the membrane material most widely used for GBR procedures is constructed of a specifically structured form of expanded polytetrafluoroethylene (e-PTFE; Gore-Tex Augmentation Material, W.L. Gore). The fluorocarbon molecule, polytetrafluoroethylene (the base chemical component of e-PTFE), cannot be chemically broken down in physiologic conditions. Additionally, safety of e-PTFE has been established by extensive biocompatibility testing and a long history of safe and effective use in vascular and soft tissue prostheses.[8]

It may be possible to develop safe and effective degradable GBR membranes. However, degradable materials have specific biocompatibility issues that must be addressed in membrane design, and they present additional concerns with regard to patient safety and membrane function. The breakdown products released by degradable materials into the surrounding tissue of the host can be both chemical and physical in nature, and each form can affect cellular and systemic response. In addition to the primary breakdown products, any contaminants or additives within a degradable device (such as platicizers incorporated to improve handling) will also enter the host. It is necessary to identify all substances that result from degradation and understand the potential local and systemic effects these products will have on the patient.

The synthetic polymer materials most often proposed for use as GBR membranes (polylactic acid and polyglycolic acid) degrade by the process of hydrolysis, with the end point being chemical substances common to normal metabolic processes.[9] However, during the process of hydrolytic degradation, these materials lose mechanical integrity and break up into fragments. The physical nature and quantity of these fragments can have a significant effect on local tissue response (Fig 4-2), which can lead to actual bone resorption.[10] Therefore, not only must the end product(s) of degradation be benign, but the biocompatibility characteristics of the intermediate breakdown products must be taken into account and controlled in material design.

Biocompatibility and Immunologic Response

It can be argued that any host reaction to a foreign material is a response of the immune system.[6] However, the immunologic response of primary concern for patient safety involves direct or indirect hypersensitivity to the implanted material. As a result, potential antigenic responses must be considered in the selection of materials for an implantable device. Synthetic materials used in implantable devices are not normally regarded as potent antigens, although some of the components of certain polymers, usually residual monomers, can evoke delayed hypersensitivity reactions in some patients.[11]

A common misconception is that all collagen-based biomaterials are identical in composition. In fact, the manner in which donor collagen is processed has a significant effect on device structure, mechanical properties, immunogenic potential, and degradation time. A primary concern, given the protein composition of collagen, is the potential for systemic immunologic reactions, particularly hypersensitization and cross-reactivity.[12] The immunogenic potential of collagen materials can be minimized by reducing telopeptide residues or by cross-linking, but appropriate animal and clinical immunogenicity testing is necessary to ensure patient safety.

Biocompatibility and Osteogenesis

The general function of a membrane used for GBR therapy is to create an environment that will allow normal healing processes to form bone in a defined region. Therefore, the host-biomaterial interactions should not interfere with bone formation and maintenance to a clinically significant degree. In part, the degree to which a material may interfere with bone healing relates to the degree and extent of chronic inflammation seen with a particular material. Orthopedic[13] and oral surgery[14] literature has identified that a pronounced foreign-body reaction can result in lack of bone formation and even osteolysis. Therefore, biomaterial chemistry and structure should result in minimal foreign-body response (Fig 4-3). At the very least, any chronic inflammatory response should not extend far beyond the borders of the material, because a diffuse chronic inflammatory response may compromise bone healing.

Good bone-biomaterial interaction characteristics are also desirable. A GBR membrane that allows close adaptation of bone tissue will allow more complete fill of the space defined by the membrane and stabilization of the membrane within the overall system (Fig 4-4).

Biocompatibility and Tissue Integration

Membranes used in GBR therapy need to achieve an adequate degree of tissue integration between the connective tissue and the membrane. While this subject will be dealt with in greater detail later in this chapter, the biocompatibility characteristics of the material have an important effect on tissue integration. The capacity of a material to achieve tissue integration is determined, to a significant degree, by the nature of the cellular response to the material. The basic goal of material design is to provide an acceptable chemical composition and an appropriate material structure that will allow connective tissue ingrowth or attachment to the membrane during healing. To achieve tissue integration,

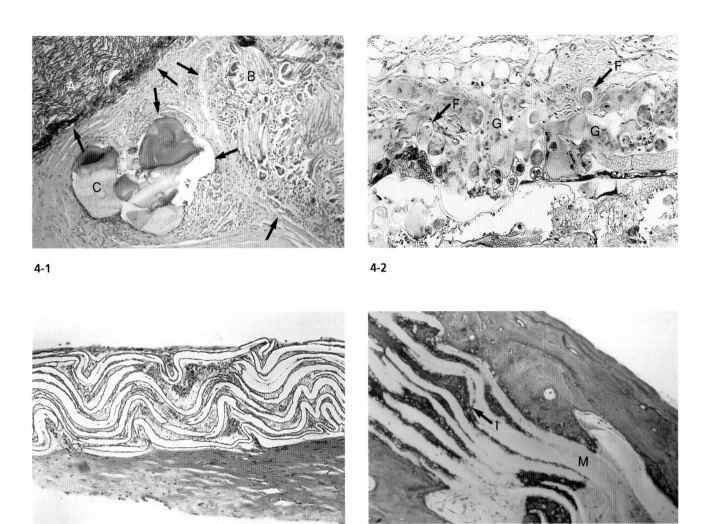

4-1

4-2

4-3

4-4

Fig 4-1 An e-PTFE vascular graft (A) and a polyethylene terapthalate vascular graft (B) have been anastamosed using polypropylene suture (C). Note the differences in the level of chronic inflammatory response to each material and the degree of fibrous capsule formation *(arrows)*. Hematoxylin and eosin stain; original magnification × 40.

Fig 4-2 Polylactide (PLA) membrane after 8 weeks of degradation in a subperiosteal site (rabbit model). Note PLA membrane fragments (F) and resultant foreign-body response characterized by multinucleate giant cells (G). Villanueva's mineralized bone stain; original magnification × 100.

Fig 4-3 Cross section of an e-PTFE membrane designed for GBR shows minimal foreign-body reaction (FBR). Minimal FBR ensures that the host-material interaction will not interfere with osteogenesis and is essential for tissue integration. Hematoxylin and eosin stain; original magnification × 40. (Clinical specimen courtesy of Dr R. Ross.)

Fig 4-4 Hard tissue response to an e-PTFE membrane designed for GBR that was used to treat a canine experimental alveolar ridge defect. Note direct bone apposition to the material (M) and ingrowth into the material interstices (I). Toluidine blue stain; original magnification × 40. (Photomicrograph courtesy of Dr R.K. Schenk.)

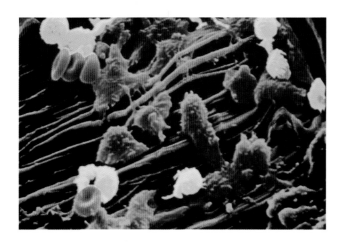

Fig 4-5 Computer-enhanced scanning electron micrograph shows fibroblasts *(blue)* adhering to the surface of an e-PTFE GBR membrane. Erythrocytes *(red)* and leukocytes *(white)* are also present. Original magnification × 4,400. (Clinical specimen and preparation courtesy of Dr P. Mattout and Dr C. Mattout.)

the foreign-body response to the material must be minimal, as a pronounced foreign-body reaction will prevent or compromise connective tissue integration and the material microstructure must be designed to encourage tissue integration. Figure 4-5 shows fibroblasts adhering to the surface of an e-PTFE membrane designed for GBR; attachment and spreading of fibroblasts are necessary precursors to deposition of collagen and subsequent tissue integration.[15]

Cell Occlusion

Membrane Structure and Cell Occlusion

In 1959 Hurley et al[16] used cellulose acetate laboratory filters and silicone rubber membranes in experimental spinal fusions. The authors' rationale, and subsequently that of Boyne[17–19] in osseous facial reconstruction, was that use of a microporous membrane would create a suitable environment for osteogenesis by excluding connective tissue cellular elements from the bone healing region. In the words of Boyne,[19] "It was hypothesized that by preventing the formation of fibrous scar tissue, greater opportunities for bone repair would be obtained." These pioneers selected membranes with cell-occlusive characteristics that would prevent the invasion of connective tissue cells originating from the soft tissue during healing.

Karring, Nyman, and coworkers published a series of papers[20–22] describing the relative contribution of different tissue types involved in periodontal wound healing. From this work it was concluded that only cells originating from the periodontal ligament possessed the potential for formation of a new connective tissue attachment (newly formed cementum with inserting collagen fibers) to a denuded root surface. In addition, this work indicated that fibrous connective tissue contact with the tooth root surface resulted in resorption of the root dentin. The investigators hypothesized that, by mechanically separating a denuded root surface from the overlying soft tissue, regeneration of the peri-odontal attachment apparatus might be possible. This hypothesis was confirmed when microporous cellulose acetate laboratory fil-ters were placed over experimentally induced periodontal defects in monkeys[23] and in a human subject.[24] The rationale for use of the membranes was to prevent undesirable tissues, in this case both fibrous connective tissue and dentogingival epithelium, from par-ticipating in healing events adjacent to the tooth root surface. Once again, the investigators selected membrane characteristics that would prevent connective tissue penetration. The term "guided tissue regeneration" (GTR) was coined from this work to describe both the biologic events and the technique of treatment employed.

Based on this pioneering research, investigators in this field have mostly selected membranes or other devices with cell-occlusive properties, regardless of material type, for regeneration of periodontal and oral osseous tissues.[25–30] Cell-occlusive mem-branes have been chosen based on the assumption that fibrous scar tissue *proliferation* is detrimental to osseous regeneration. Indeed, work by Ogiso et al[31] suggests that gingival connective tissue fibroblasts have the potential to inhibit osteogenesis in vitro.

A number of studies, however, report observations that are not readily explained by the "cell exclusion" component of classical GTR theory (ie, that fibrous connective tissue must be excluded from an area for bone formation to occur). Murray et al[32] placed "fenestrated" plastic cages on the surface of dog ilia. No details are given for the size or number of the fenestrations, but from the authors' description of the cages it is probable that these fen-estrations were macroscopic. If so, macroscopic holes would not prevent proliferation of fibrous connective tissue into the interior of the cages. Although no histology is presented in the paper, the authors reported that the interior of the cages filled with bone. Nielson et al[33] created bilateral critical-size defects (nonsponta-neously healing) in rabbit radii. They adapted a polyurethane membrane, forming a tube, to the bone ends in each experimen-tal site. Membranes were not placed over the contralateral con-trol defects. After 5 weeks of healing, the authors reported bridg-ing of the experimental defects by bone callus on the outside of the tube, whereas the space inside the tube was occupied by fibrous connective tissue. Classical GTR theory would predict the opposite result, or at the very least, that bone would not form on the outside of the membrane, where fibrous connective tissue cer-tainly had the opportunity to compete with bone formation. Linde et al[34] described formation of bone on a mature cortical bone surface when using dome-shaped e-PTFE membranes placed on the calvaria of rats. One of the membrane designs the authors utilized was a very porous form of e-PTFE (pores up to 100 μm). These membranes, which allowed connective tissue penetration through the wall thickness of the membranes, showed greater bone formation than membranes of smaller (more occlusive) pore size. The authors also reported bone formation taking place on the outside of the membranes.

Other examples of bone formation taking place without the exclusion of fibrous connective tissue are osteophyte formation associated with osteoarthritis, the dramatic results that can be obtained with distraction osteogenesis,[35] and external callus formation commonly seen with simple fracture healing.[36]

In view of this conflicting information, it appears that the biologic necessity for a fully occlusive membrane has not been clearly demonstrated and that further research is needed to fully characterize the mechanism(s) of interaction between bone and fibrous connective tissue during healing. When obtained, this information can possibly be applied to membrane design to enhance GBR membrane function.

Membrane Structure and Nutrient Transfer

It has been suggested that membranes used for bone regeneration should have porous properties that allow for the transfer of nutrient fluids and gases. For example, Boyne[19] states "... the [cellulose acetate] filter provided for ample transfer of tissue fluids to the graft sites." This concept is based on the rationale that nutrient transport across the membrane may improve the environment for bone regeneration. Indeed, some evidence suggests an important role for transport of nutrients across a membrane. Hurley et al[16] included membranes composed of nonporous silicone rubber in a study of experimental spinal fusions. The sites with the nonporous membranes failed to heal with bone formation. In contrast, the microporous cellulose acetate membrane sites healed completely with bone.

While nutrient transfer across a GBR membrane may be an important consideration, there are many unanswered questions regarding this issue. For example, for substances to cross the membrane there must be a physicochemical driving force for diffusion, probably determined by concentration gradients. In what direction would the concentration gradients be established? Would the concentration gradients be of sufficient magnitude to result in diffusion of physiologically significant quantities of nutrient substances? Across what distances could significant quantities of substances be diffused in physiologic conditions? What membrane structure(s) would allow diffusion of clinically important substances and yet meet the other functions required of a GBR membrane (such as protection from bacterial challenge)? Clearly this issue contains fertile ground for further research. It is also likely that other factors, such as an adequate vascular source origi- nating from the parent bone and an adequate source of osteogenic cells,[36] may be of equal or greater influence in the regenerative outcome.

Does this mean that GBR membranes should not be occlusive and could be modified to perform more adequately in other func- tions such as tissue integration (ie, be more porous)? As always, it is necessary to evaluate device design in the full context of clinical requirements, as illustrated in the following section.

It is important to note that the "cell exclusion" component of classical GTR theory has not, by any means, been disproved. Until experimental evidence proves otherwise, the most prudent approach to membrane design is to utilize adequate cell-occlusive properties that have shown predictable clinical performance.

Membrane Structure and Bacterial Protection

Cell-occlusive membrane properties perform an additional crucial function. Obtaining and maintaining soft tissue closure simplifies the treatment course for any given case. However, in the context of alveolar bone regeneration, the anatomic, mechanical, and technical realities of clinical therapy virtually assure that some membranes will become exposed to the oral environment in the course of treatment. Membrane exposure leads to the possibility of bacterial challenge and resulting acute inflammation that may be detrimental to osteogenesis,[37] but does not necessarily result in failure of the procedure. Therefore, the membrane must provide some degree of protection from bacterial challenge in the event of exposure (Figs 4-6a to c). A membrane with porous characteris- tics that allow bacterial penetration into the regenerative space (Fig 4-7) may compromise the regenerative result.

There are several possible ways of addressing this situation from a material design standpoint, but this discussion will focus on fac- tors involving membrane structure. Specifically, occlusive proper- ties must be incorporated into the membrane structure, and there must be an adequate degree of tissue integration between the membrane and the surrounding tissue in order to form a biologic seal (see the following discussion on tissue integration).

The structure of the most commonly used GBR membrane designed specifically for alveolar ridge regeneration has an inner (central) portion that is occlusive to cellular penetration (Fig 4-8). In addition to providing stiffness (see discussion on spacemaking), this occlusive portion of the membrane is designed to serve as a barrier against invasion of fibrous connective tissue and to pro- vide some degree of protection from bacterial challenge for the defect region (Fig 4-9). The outer, more porous portion of the membrane is designed to ingrow and attach to surrounding tissue, form a biologic seal, and prevent bacteria from tracking

Bacterial protection in the event of membrane exposure.

Figs 4-6a to c

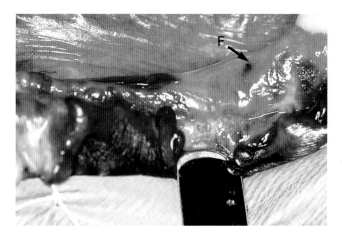

4-6a

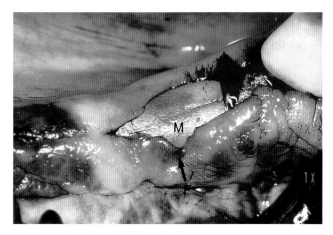

4-6b

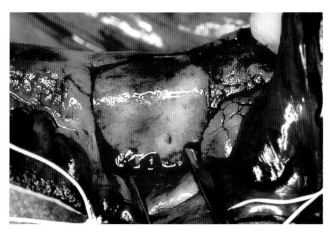

4-6c

Fig 4-6a   Fistula (F) 25 days after membrane placement in a canine experimental GBR model. The fistula formed as a result of a suture line dehiscence and could be probed to the underlying e-PTFE GBR membrane. The initial dehiscence occurred 4 days postoperatively; daily antimicrobial control measures helped maintain clinical stability.

Fig 4-6b   Surgical re-entry of the site. The e-PTFE membrane, designed for GBR, covered a surgically created defect approximately 7 × 7 × 10 mm. Note the position of the fistula (F) relative to the membrane (M), which is still in place.

Fig 4-6c   Appearance of the site after membrane removal revealed no evidence of bacteria-induced inflammation in the tissue underneath the membrane after 21 days of exposure. A thin layer of what appeared to be fibrous connective tissue interfaced with the membrane, and residual coagulum (C) in the defect could be seen under this layer.

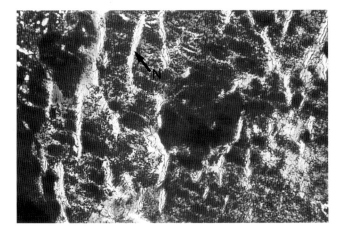

4-7

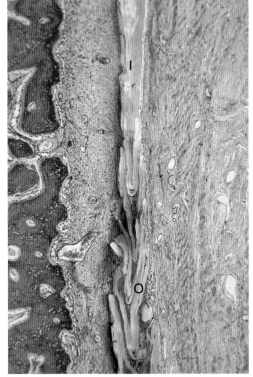

4-8

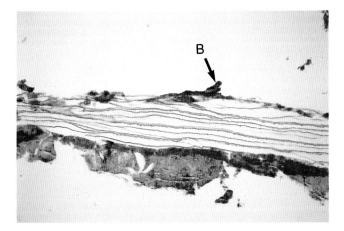

4-9

Fig 4-7 Cross section of a moderately porous (pores > 25 μm) e-PTFE laboratory filter that was used to treat a periodontal defect and became exposed to the oral environment. Note invasion of the material interstices by Gram-positive bacterial colonies *(purple)*. N indicates PTFE nodes. Brown-Bren stain for bacteria; original magnification × 100.

Fig 4-8 Two-part e-PTFE membrane designed for GBR. Note the lack of cellular penetration into the inner occlusive portion (I) and the ingrowth of tissue into the outer porous portion (O). Basic fuchsin stain; original magnification × 16. (Photomicrograph courtesy of Dr R.K. Schenk.)

Fig 4-9 Occlusive properties of an e-PTFE membrane designed for GBR. Note bacteria on material surface (B) and lack of bacterial penetration through the membrane structure. Brown-Bren stain for bacteria; original magnification × 40. (Clinical specimen courtesy of Dr R. Valentine.)

around the edge of the membrane. Although this outer portion of the membrane is not fully occlusive to the penetration of fibrous connective tissue, Warrer et al[37] have shown that there is no qualitative difference between the regenerative capability of this more porous material structure and that of the highly occlusive inner portion.

The specific requirements for bacterial protection (occlusiveness) of a GBR membrane are not completely understood, and further research will allow improvements in membrane design and performance. Certainly the porosity of a membrane can be characterized by various testing methods (see tissue integration); however, performance must ultimately be determined by clinical testing.

Maintenance of a stable relationship between the integrated tissue and the membrane, in the event of exposure, is dependent on a number of factors. A biomaterial integrated with fibrous connective tissue and partially exposed to the oral cavity exists in a hostile and challenging environment. Moisture, mechanical stress, and inevitable contamination by bacteria make maintenance of a stable, integrated relationship between the membrane and tissue very tenuous. Despite the best of material designs, membrane exposure is a situation that must be monitored closely, and managed carefully, by both the clinician and the patient.

Tissue Integration

Clinical Benefits

The phenomena of *ingrowth* and *surface bonding* of tissue to a biomaterial are termed *integration*. Surface and microstructural characteristics are primarily responsible for determining whether ingrowth or surface bonding of tissue occurs during healing. For example, titanium "osseointegrated" implants appear to demonstrate surface bonding, while porous coated hip prostheses allow bony ingrowth and may also exhibit surface bonding. The clinical benefits of GBR membranes that have the capacity to integrate with surrounding tissues are a result of a more mechanically stable (and therefore predictable) wound healing environment and the potential for protection of the coagulum-filled space should the membrane become exposed. While tissue integration appears to be necessary for optimal performance of a GBR membrane, chemical and structural properties that encourage tissue integration must be balanced with the overall functional requirements of alveolar ridge regeneration (eg, the need for cell-occlusive properties).

Fig 4-10 Photomicrograph showing the stable relationship between the tooth root surface, viable cementum, inserting crestal fibers, and epithelium. The apical extent of the epithelium is determined by the location of intact crestal fibers *(arrow)*. Hematoxylin and eosin stain; original magnification × 10. (Photomicrograph courtesy of Dr R. Caffesse.)

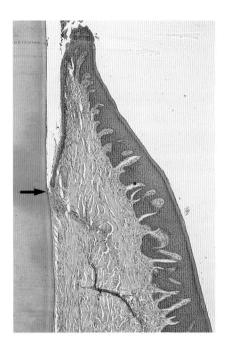

Tissue Integration and Epithelial Inhibition

Winter[38] observed that, in a periodontally healthy condition, sulcular epithelium forms a stable seal at the tooth–epithelium–gingival crestal fiber junction (Fig 4-10). When the gingival crestal fibers are broken down by disease, the epithelium migrates rapidly over connective tissue abutting the tooth to the level of intact inserting fibers, thus forming a periodontal pocket. Winter proposed that gingival crestal fibers, inserting into cementum on the tooth surface, create a barrier that inhibits epithelial migration. He termed this phenomenon "contact inhibition."

Winter also found that the phenomenon of contact inhibition could be duplicated with transepithelial biomaterials if the materials were adequately porous and allowed ingrowth and attachment of connective tissue. He concluded that connective tissue ingrowth and attachment to a porous biomaterial can provide the same function as collagen fibers inserting into the cementum of a tooth. Without connective tissue attachment, the epithelium migrates rapidly around the implant, forming a sinus tract that isolates the foreign body (implant), eventually resulting in extrusion of the material from the tissue.[39] In addition, lack of a stable, integrated situation at the epithelium–connective tissue–biomaterial interface leaves the site prone to bacterial invasion and infection.

The phenomenon of contact inhibition has been shown to be important in the functioning of transgingival biomaterials. To illustrate this, small silicone buttons were made with "skirts" of an extremely porous and highly organized e-PTFE material (Fig 4-11a). Expanded polytetrafluoroethylene is a complex, organized three-dimensional matrix of nodes and interconnecting fibrils that can be produced in a variety of porosities and structures. The e-PTFE material used in this study was characterized by large nodes of PTFE spaced 100 to 300 μm apart (Fig 4-11b). (The distance between nodes, or internodal distance, is one measure of the porosity of e-PTFE materials.) Ninety percent of the material volume was porous to allow for connective tissue ingrowth.

The e-PTFE skirt was measured for density and evaluated by scanning electron micrography, and the porosity was quantitatively characterized by measuring pore size and distribution (porosimetry). Typical structural characteristics for the material are shown in Table 4-1.

Thirty-six buttons with these e-PTFE skirts were placed in edentulous ridges in dog mandibles using midline crestal incisions, so that the silicone buttons protruded through the attached gingiva and the e-PTFE skirt rested on the alveolar crest beneath the gingiva (Fig 4-11c). Eight silicone buttons with nonporous silicone skirts

Fig 4-11a Silicone transgingival buttons (B) with attached, highly porous (>100 to 300-μm pores) e-PTFE skirts (S).

Fig 4-11b Scanning electron micrograph cross section of highly porous e-PTFE skirt. Large nodes (N) of PTFE are spaced 100 to 300 μm apart and are connected by thin fibrils (F). The skirt is 90% air by volume to allow for connective tissue ingrowth.

Fig 4-11c Buttons with attached skirts of highly porous e-PTFE are implanted in edentulous areas of dogs in such a way that the silicone button (B) protrudes through the gingiva and the e-PTFE skirt rests on the mandibular ridge beneath the attached gingiva (3 months after placement).

Fig 4-11d Photomicrograph of tissue adjacent to a button with attached nonporous silicone skirt. Arrows indicate the interface between the silicone skirt (button and skirt lost during sectioning). There is no evidence of tissue attachment to the nonporous skirt, and the collagen fibers are oriented parallel to the silicone surface encapsulating the implant. Masson's trichrome stain; original magnification × 10.

Fig 4-11e Photomicrograph of highly porous e-PTFE skirt and adjacent tissue. Note the organized channels of connective tissue (C) ingrown into the interstices of the e-PTFE material (N = PTFE nodes) and lack of encapsulation response at the skirt interface (SI). The open space between epithelial surfaces (E) was occupied by the transgingival silicone button (lost during sectioning). Epithelial migration has stopped at the skirt-button junction (SB). Masson's trichrome stain; original magnification × 10.

Phenomenon of epithelial ("contact") inhibition.

Figs   4-11a to e

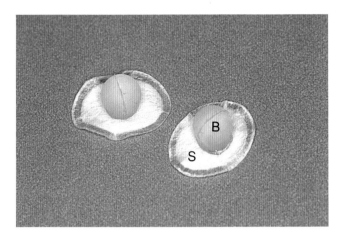

4-11a

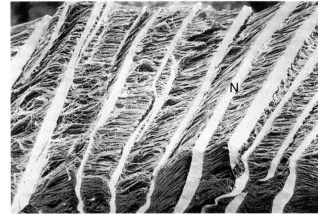

4-11b

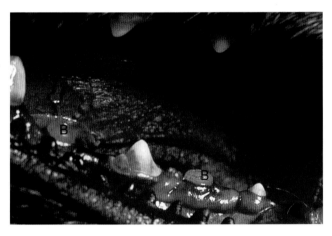

4-11c

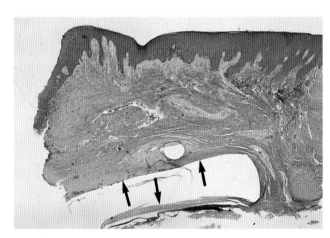

4-11d

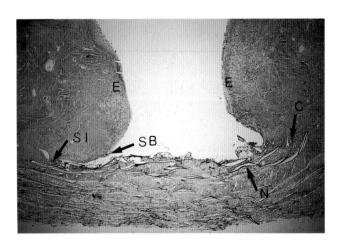

4-11e

Table 4-1 *Structural Characteristics of Experimental e-PTFE Membranes Attached to Silicone Rubber Buttons**

Bubble point (psi)	Mean flow (psi)	100% flow (psi)	Fibril length (μm)
0.2	1.1	2.4	204

*Bubble point distribution describes the range of porosity encountered within a given material when a wetting agent (ethanol in these tests) is driven out of the material by increasing air pressure. It is derived from the bubble point pressure (the "largest pore" in the material), the mean flow pressure ("half" the available porosity), and the 100% flow value ("all" available porosity). These values are relative and can be used to compare materials of different structures. Fibril length represents the average distance between "nodes" of the e-PTFE. Measurements were made from one node to the next, parallel to the orientation of the fibrils.

were implanted as controls. The buttons were harvested for histologic observation at either 1 or 3 months. The test buttons remained in the dogs without becoming exposed or infected. There was no gingival recession, flap necrosis, or exposure of the underlying e-PTFE. Tissue appearance was normal. The control buttons with nonporous silicone skirts were exfoliated within the first 2 weeks following surgery. Gingival tissue appeared to recede or slough away from the buttons and underlying silicone skirts.

Histologically in the control buttons, tissue attachment or ingrowth had failed to occur along the silicone skirt. Collagen fibrils were aligned parallel to the skirt and formed a dense capsule (Fig 4-11d). Gingival epithelium had apparently migrated along the tissue bed adjacent to the silicone skirts until the buttons were extruded. In the test buttons, the porous e-PTFE skirt appeared well ingrown with organized channels of connective tissue. Epithelial migration had stopped at the e-PTFE skirt interface (Fig 4-11e). It appeared that ingrowth and attachment stabilized the wound and prevented the gingival flaps from sloughing or receding, while the same organized connective tissue ingrowth also limited the migration of epithelium (pocketing) adjacent to the implant.

Different e-PTFE membrane porosities have been tested to determine the ideal porosity range for tissue integration, wound stabilization, and contact inhibition. Tissue integration into e-PTFE membrane structures was graded according to histologic evaluation that ranked tissue attachment and percent of collagen ingrowth. This ranking was then compared to membrane porosity characteristics to determine the relationship between porosity and tissue integration. The structure of e-PTFE is characterized by a highly oriented structure of nodes interconnected with fibrils. The three-dimensional matrix of e-PTFE presents an acceptable matrix for tissue ingrowth as a result of the specific porous structure, mechanical properties (such as elastic modulus), and the characteristic surface chemistry of PTFE, which has a very low surface energy (25 dynes/cm^2). Consequently, the porous characteristics of other membranes (eg, polyesters or polypeptides with machined, dissoluted, or woven porosities) cannot be directly compared to e-PTFE. To determine the effectiveness of other regenerative membranes, extensive in vitro tests and in vivo trials must be performed in appropriate animal and clinical models examining porosity, chemical composition, tissue integration, and consequential wound stabilization and contact inhibition.

Periodontal research with membranes that do not have the structural capacity for tissue integration has resulted in membrane exposure, rapid epithelial pocketing, and resultant tissue inflammation and poor regenerative results (Figs 4-12a to c). A number of periodontal studies have been conducted with both resorbable and nonresorbable membranes that did not possess tissue integration characteristics. Card et al[40] described the clinical observations of collagen membranes used in a naturally occurring periodontal disease beagle dog model. The authors state, "… in several areas the membrane was no doubt exfoliated. This led to a lower mean value for new attachment. Most importantly, the amount of new attachment gained in these studies was highly variable…." Warrer et al,[41] using polylactic acid and polyurethane membranes, concluded that "… the GTR procedure is sensitive with respect to the characteristics of the membrane which is used. The ability to prevent or retard epithelial migration along its surface seems to be a fundamental requirement."

In contrast, membranes that are designed to allow for tissue integration appear to provide the capacity to inhibit or slow the migration and pocketing of gingival epithelium in periodontal regeneration or in the event of membrane exposure (Fig 4-13). Caffesse et al[42] used an e-PTFE membrane designed for tissue integration to treat naturally occurring periodontitis in beagle dogs and found that the proliferation of the junctional epithelium was halted, with most of the marginal seals being established by a short junctional epithelium. Kon et al[43] compared an e-PTFE membrane, designed for periodontal regeneration and tissue integration, with a woven polyester (polylactic acid/polyglycolic acid copolymer) mesh, designed for reconstruction of soft tissue defects, in a surgically created, chronic periodontal defect model in mongrel dogs. They found greater levels of new cementum formation with the e-PTFE group compared to the polyester mesh group. The e-PTFE group also showed formation of a "short junctional epithelium."

Any membrane used in alveolar ridge GBR is at risk for exposure to the oral environment, whether because of the membrane's proximity to adjacent teeth, the presence of an overlying incision or tissue dehiscence, insufficient soft tissue to allow primary closure, or unintended trauma. A membrane designed for optimal function must, therefore, have characteristics allowing for the establishment of a stable epithelium–connective tissue–membrane

Membrane lacking capacity for tissue integration.

Figs 4-12a to c

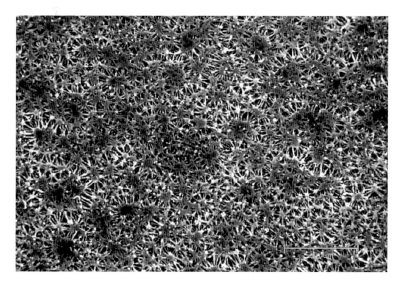

4-12a

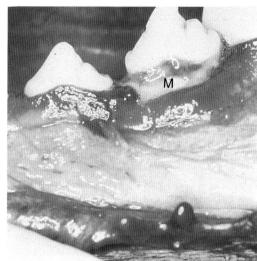

4-12b

Fig 4-12a Scanning electron micrograph of the surface of a small-pore (<1 μm) e-PTFE membrane with structural characteristics designed to prevent tissue integration.

Fig 4-12b Small-pore (<1 μm) e-PTFE membrane (M) used to treat a surgically created periodontal defect in a canine model (28 days after membrane placement). Lack of tissue integration resulted in soft tissue recession and inflammation.

Fig 4-12c Photomicrograph of a surgically created canine periodontal defect treated with small-pore (<1 μm) e-PTFE membrane that showed lack of tissue integration with resultant recession, membrane exposure (M), debris impaction (D), and soft tissue inflammation. Hematoxylin and eosin stain; original magnification × 2.5.

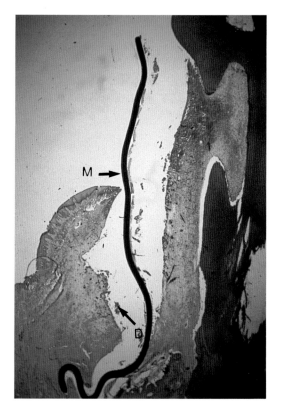

4-12c

Fig 4-13 An e-PTFE membrane used to treat a surgically created periodontal defect in a monkey shows good tissue integration 3 months after placement. Epithelial migration (E) has stopped at the coronal margin of the porous structure (P), which is ingrown with connective tissue. Note the base of the defect (D) and regeneration of periodontal structures beneath the membrane. Hematoxylin and eosin stain; original magnification × 2.5.

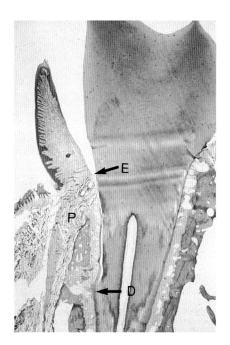

junction in the event of membrane exposure. This is accomplished by providing a membrane microstructure that will encourage connective tissue ingrowth and attachment (see Fig 4-3), resulting in oriented gingival connective tissue integration that will inhibit or slow epithelial migration (Fig 4-13).

Tissue Integration and Wound Stability

Direct bone healing (bone healing without a cartilage precursor) is dependent on establishing, at least initially, a mechanically stable environment.[36] Although appropriate levels of mechanical stress are necessary for the maintenance and functional remodeling of bone,[44] disruptive stress early in the healing process may prevent bone healing and result in scar formation.

Guided bone regeneration therapy not only involves osseous healing events taking place beneath the membrane, but also includes management of, and healing events related to, the soft tissue. Wound stabilization can dramatically affect soft tissue healing. A deep skin wound that is not stabilized and supported by suturing or other means will heal if kept clean and infection-free, but the healing time will be greatly extended and possibly result in heavy scarring. Without proper attention given to the surgical approach and the interactions of the membrane with the soft tissue, therapeutic results may be compromised or the procedure may fail completely.

Nonporous, nontextured biomaterials, implanted in soft tissue, generally exhibit the formation of a fibrous connective tissue capsule, where there is no attachment of the tissue to the material, and the collagen fibers of the capsule are oriented parallel to the material surface.[45] Also, mechanical stress causing relative movement at the interface between the implanted material and the tissue can result in thickening of the capsule and can lead to pronounced chronic inflammation.[46] Hurley et al[16] attributed the formation of a thick, fibrous connective tissue capsule, and incomplete bone formation adjacent to silicone sheets used to treat experimental spinal fusions, to the lack of material porosity and, therefore, limited diffusion of nutrients into the defect regions. However, it is possible that at least part of the reason for capsule formation was the normal cellular and tissue response to the smooth surface of the material and relative movement at the tissue-silicone interface.

Integration of a membrane material with the surrounding tissue helps to provide the stability necessary for both osseous and soft tissue healing. Claffey et al[47] showed that a very porous (>100-μm pores) e-PTFE membrane that allowed tissue integration provided mechanical support for the gingival tissues during periodontal wound healing. Haney et al[48] have demonstrated experimentally that an e-PTFE membrane designed to allow connective tissue integration provides wound stabilization during periodontal wound healing. They found that when adequate space was available

Fig 4-14a   An e-PTFE membrane designed for alveolar ridge GBR, composed of two portions with different structural properties (I = inner portion; O = outer portion).

Fig 4-14b   Cross section scanning electron micrograph of the inner portion. This structure is relatively stiff, for a greater degree of spacemaking ability, and occlusive (limited interstitial space).

Fig 4-14c   Cross section scanning electron micrograph of the outer portion. This structure is more supple, to allow adaptation to bone contours, and porous (average pore size 20 to 25 μm). Note PTFE nodes (N) and interstitial spaces (I).

Fig 4-14d   Inner portion (I) shows minimal tissue attachment and is occlusive for protection from fibrous connective tissue and bacterial invasion. Outer portion (O) is porous to allow tissue integration for wound stability and to limit epithelial pocketing in the event of membrane exposure. Separation of the tissue from the inner portion occurred during histologic processing due to the minimal degree of attachment to the occlusive structure. Mallory's trichrome stain; original magnification × 10. (Clinical specimen courtesy of Dr R. Ross.)

Fig 4-14e   Outer structure of an e-PTFE membrane designed for GBR. Note the invasion of the interstitial spaces of the membrane by fibrous connective tissue (I). N indicates PTFE nodes. Basic fuchsin stain; original magnification × 40. (Photomicrograph courtesy of Dr R.K. Schenk.)

Two-part design of e-PTFE membrane promotes tissue integration.

Figs 4-14a to e

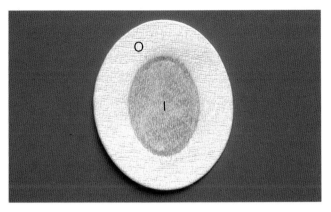

4-14a

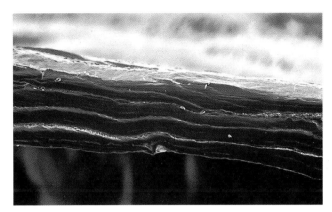

4-14b

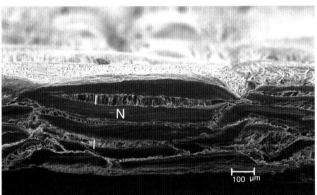

4-14c

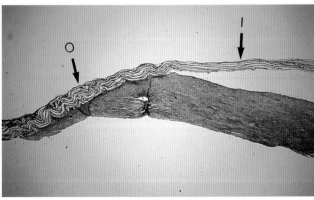
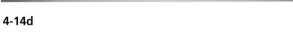

4-14d

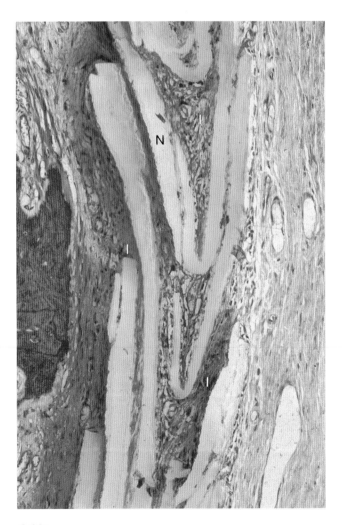

4-14e

between the membrane and tooth root surface, significantly more bone regeneration occurred at the membrane-treated sites than at the nonmembrane control sites. The improved bone regeneration was due, in part, to the mechanically stable wound healing situation. Additional wound stability can be provided by mechanically securing the membrane to the hard tissue.[4,49]

The two-part design of the most commonly used GBR membrane (Figs 4-14a to c) incorporates structural features that allow and encourage tissue integration. Specifically, the outer portion of the e-PTFE membrane has internodal distances of 20 to 25 μm (Fig 4-14c) and has a surface structure that encourages connective tissue attachment. Experimental and clinical experience has shown that this structure allows ingrowth of connective tissue into the material interstices and attachment of the material to the connective tissue (Figs 4-14d and e; see also Fig 4-3). In addition, the tissue integration characteristics of this material are, in part, responsible for the protection provided in clinical situations where membranes have been exposed to the oral environment.[50,51]

Spacemaking

Importance of Creating and Maintaining a Space During GBR

The term "bone regeneration" implies that, during treatment, a specific volume of space, preferably in a specific geometry, is filled with viable bone tissue to restore function and/or esthetics. In GBR therapy, this space and geometry are defined by the borders of the parent bone and the overlying membrane. This space and geometry must be created and maintained for an adequate period of time during healing for acceptable therapeutic results.

Haney et al[48] have shown that bone regeneration in membrane-treated, surgically produced periodontal defects in dogs is a function of the amount of space available between the membrane and the tooth surface. Although the authors do not give a minimum amount of space necessary to allow bone regeneration, the results suggest such a limit. Numerous other studies dating back to the 1950s have identified the importance of creating a protected space during GBR procedures.[1,2,25,32,52,53]

To create and maintain adequate space volume and geometry, a GBR membrane not only must support its own weight but must resist the pressure exerted by overlying tissue and external forces such as mastication. Therefore, the spacemaking characteristics of a GBR membrane can be defined in terms of the membrane's ability to resist collapse.

Membrane collapse results in elimination of the necessary space (Figs 4-15a to c) and, given the occlusive nature of GBR membranes, the device may effectively prevent regeneration. For example, Kohavi et al[54] closely adapted e-PTFE membranes to the surfaces of surgically created alveolar ridge defects in dogs to ensure that spontaneous regeneration would not occur. They found that the membranes prevented spontaneous regeneration of the bone and that the contour of the bone surface was determined by the contour of the membranes.

Membrane Characteristics and Spacemaking

The resistance to collapse of a GBR membrane is determined largely by the material stiffness. As a result, it would appear that a very stiff membrane would be optimal for GBR procedures. However, the spacemaking function (stiffness) of a membrane must be balanced with the capacity to adapt the membrane to the contours of the adjacent bone and to minimize the tendency for the material to perforate the delicate soft tissues of the oral cavity—requirements that call for softer, more flexible membrane characteristics.

In the most commonly used membrane in GBR therapy the inner portion is stiff relative to the outer, more supple portion (see Fig- 4-14a). The stiffer inner portion is designed to have a greater degree of spacemaking capability and is intended to be placed directly over the area where space maintenance is most critical. The more supple outer portion is designed to allow greater ease in conforming to the bone contours and to minimize the potential for mucosal perforation. Future membrane research will focus, in part, on the development of membranes that are significantly stiffer than those currently available and, at the same time, conform to adjacent anatomy.[55]

Membrane Characteristics and Spacemaking Duration

Woven bone formation begins at the surfaces of the parent bone[36,56] and proceeds toward the interior of the defect. The rate of woven bone formation is dependent on the rates of revascularization and osteoblast recruitment.[36] Therefore, the distance to be spanned by bone regeneration will determine the time that the membrane must remain in place and functionally intact.

Space maintenance throughout the necessary healing period is dependent on maintenance of the mechanical and physical integrity of the membrane. An inert material (nondegradable), with sufficient strength to maintain mechanical and structural integrity in the face of normal mechanical challenge, will maintain full spacemaking capabilities throughout the necessary healing period (Fig 4-15c).

In contrast, degradable materials do not degrade instantaneously, but rather over a period of time and at rates determined by a number of factors. The degradable materials mentioned thus far (collagen, polylactic acid, and polyglycolic acid) generally begin to lose mechanical strength, and therefore spacemaking capability, soon after they are implanted.[9] Therefore, degradable membranes with different mechanical and physical degradation rates may be required for defects with different morphology. In addition, a degradable membrane that is designed to maintain the mechanical characteristics required for adequate bone healing may not be completely degraded for many months after loss of structural integrity. Incomplete material degradation may present additional risks for infection at the dental implant site when communication between the oral cavity and the material is established at implant abutment placement.

Techniques for Additional Membrane Support

With current membrane technology, the ability to create and maintain a space adjacent to a bone surface is dependent, in part, on the mechanical characteristics of the membrane and on the morphology of the adjacent bone. In situations where membrane stiffness and bone morphology are inadequate, clinical techniques and adjunctive materials or devices have been developed that provide support for the membrane.[3,19,53,57,58] These important topics are discussed elsewhere in this book.

Fig 4-15a   Schematic diagram of spacemaking (good resistance to collapse) and non-spacemaking (poor resistance to collapse) membranes showing the space-eliminating effects of membrane collapse.

Fig 4-15b   An e-PTFE GBR membrane (M) was used to treat a large (10 × 10 × 10 mm) experimental alveolar ridge defect. This membrane partially collapsed under pressure of overlying tissue, resulting in reduction of the space (S) available for osseous regeneration (2 months after membrane placement). Basic fuchsin stain; original magnification × 2. (Photomicrograph courtesy of Dr R.K. Schenk.)

Fig 4-15c   An e-PTFE membrane (M) reinforced to provide good resistence-to-collapse characteristics. Note the original defect surface (D), new bone (NB), and maintenance by the membrane of the arched shape of the alveolar ridge. A stainless steel mini-screw was used to fix the membrane to the bone (2 months after membrane placement). Toluidine blue stain; original magnification × 2. (Photomicrograph courtesy of Dr R.K. Schenk.)

Membrane resistance to collapse.   *Figs 4-15a to c*

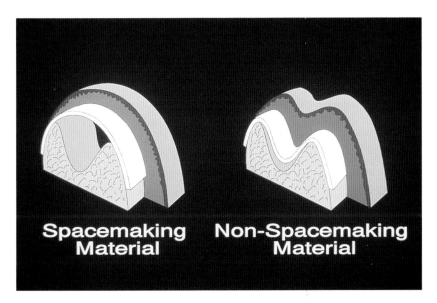

4-15a

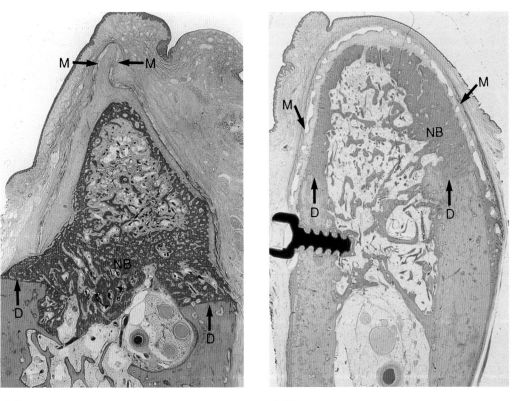

4-15b   **4-15c**

Clinical Manageability

Because membranes are an integral part of the overall GBR procedure, membrane design must take clinical requirements into account.

Clinical manageability of a GBR membrane is determined largely by the ease of surgical manipulation and postoperative management. Optimal membrane design requires minimal difficulty in operative handling to allow the clinician to achieve proper membrane placement. The duration of surgery and postoperative recovery and the impact of postoperative complications are also important considerations. Ultimately, clinical manageability influences the success and efficacy of a regenerative procedure; it can only be measured by compiling a diverse and significant number of long-term observations from both clinicians and patients.

Membrane Characteristics and Clinical Handling

Membranes used for GBR must undergo a series of physical manipulations. They are cut, shaped, and sometimes fixed in place with sutures or screws. The time and skill needed to perform regenerative osseous surgery depends, in part, on the defect treated. But regardless of the surgical site, regenerative membranes must be designed to facilitate placement and postoperative treatment. Although a variety of configurations may facilitate membrane placement (Fig 4-16), each case is unique and trimming of a membrane to the appropriate shape is often required. Therefore, a GBR membrane should be easily trimmed and manipulated without cumbersome handling and without fraying or fragmenting.

If all bone surfaces were flat, any two-dimensional membrane could be shaped to cover an osseous defect. However, every clinical situation requiring restoration of bone presents a unique three-dimensional morphology and membranes currently used in GBR therapy are, for practical purposes, two-dimensional. In more complex anatomic situations, adaptation of a two-dimensional membrane to a three-dimensional structure can be technically demanding, requiring much patience and skill on the part of the clinician. A GBR membrane must have some stiffness or have enough "memory" to be spacemaking; however, it must also conform to the bony contours (Figs 4-17a and b) without memory characteristics that force it to spring back to its original shape and possibly perforate delicate mucosal tissue. In addition to limiting the possibility for postoperative complications, anecdotal evidence suggests that better adaptation of e-PTFE membranes to the bone surface surrounding the defect results in more complete osseous regeneration.[3]

Membrane Structure and Postoperative Management

In addition to the biologic need for a GBR membrane to maintain structural integrity during healing, the membrane must also maintain its structure in the event it must be removed. Whether as a natural step in second-stage surgery or because postoperative complications indicate removal, structural or mechanical integrity ensures that the membrane can be completely removed without fragmentation (Fig 4-18). In this situation, a nondegradable membrane with appropriate mechanical strength and tissue integration characteristics will allow minimal (although not the complete absence of) difficulty in removal. Degradable membranes that have lost all or part of their mechanical strength may be difficult to remove completely. Retained membrane fragments may become the foci for further complications.

In the literature, regenerative membrane exposure is occasionally implicated in compromised osteogenic results.[37] In cases of membrane exposure, it is necessary to clearly identify the causative factors involved with compromised results. The term "exposure" indicates direct communication between the membrane and the environment of the oral cavity. Exposure results in at least a portion of the material being contaminated by bacteria. Compromised osteogenesis, however, is not a direct result of membrane exposure, but rather the induction of acute inflammation resulting from bacterial challenge in the regenerative space. With appropriate membrane structural characteristics (occlusiveness and tissue integration) and proper monitoring and care by the clinician and patient, exposure and bacterial contamination can be limited to the external surface of the membrane and the procedure can be successful.[50,51]

Conceptually, degradable membranes should simplify clinical management by eliminating the need for surgical removal. However, it is likely that degradable materials will encounter situations that require material removal. Figure 4-19 illustrates a synthetic degradable membrane material tested in periodontal defects in dogs. Nine synthetic degradable membranes of this type were placed over surgically created Class II furcation defects in nine dogs. Full soft tissue coverage of the membranes was obtained. All of the degradable membranes became exposed between 6 and 20 days after placement. Two of these membranes were exfoliated, and the remaining membranes had to be removed because of significant inflammation and, in some cases, soft tissue necrosis. It is possible that the tightly woven structure of the material did not allow integration with adjacent tissues. These sites showed significant recession, secondary pocket formation, and the opportunity for bacteria and food debris to access the pocket. In addition to these clinical sequelae, at later times the membranes were difficult to remove due to loss of structural integrity. In this instance, the bioabsorbable feature that was intended to facilitate clinical management may actually have been a hindrance.

Fig 4-16   Three configurations of two-part e-PTFE membranes allow GBR therapy for a wide range of alveolar ridge defects.

Fig 4-17a   Localized ridge augmentation using an e-PTFE membrane (M) supported by autogenous bone grafts (G).

Fig 4-17b   Note how the membrane has been cut and overlapped *(arrows)* to allow adaptation to the curve of the mandibular arch. (Clinical photographs courtesy of Dr D. Buser.)

Fig 4-18   Clinical removal of an e-PTFE GBR membrane (M). The membrane has been elevated from the bone surface (B) but not yet completely removed. The membrane must have sufficient structural integrity to allow complete removal. Ease of removal must be balanced with the requirement for tissue integration. (Clinical photograph courtesy of Dr S. Jovanovic.)

Fig 4-19   Degradable woven polyester membrane (M) was used to treat a surgically created periodontal defect in a canine model. Note extensive recession of soft tissue possibly due to lack of tissue integration with the material structure (30 days after membrane placement).

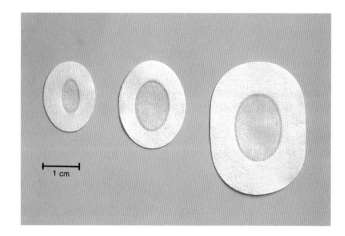

4-16

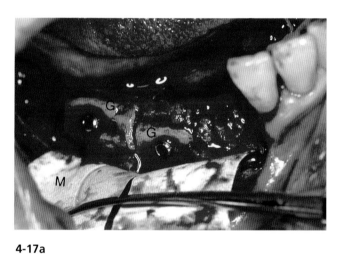

4-17a

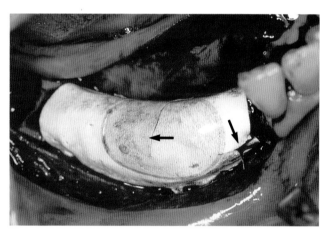

4-17b

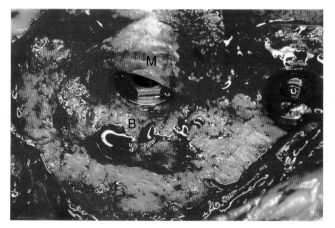

4-18

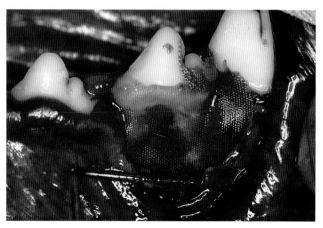

4-19

Summary

Classic GBR theory is not complex in concept: Mechanically prevent undesirable tissues from participating in the healing process in a defined area adjacent to a bone surface and osteogenesis will occur within the space. However, a membrane specifically designed to function at an acceptable clinical level in alveolar ridge GBR must incorporate a number of features that address biologic, mechanical, and clinical use requirements in addition to serving as a cell-occlusive barrier. These requirements and the membrane design solutions have been developed through extensive material and clinical testing.

The biocompatibility characteristics of membranes used for GBR therapy of the alveolar process should not present long- or short-term safety concerns for the patient. In addition, the material must illicit minimal foreign-body response during the period the membrane is in place and have biocompatibility characteristics that encourage connective tissue integration.

Some experimental evidence suggests that fibrous connective proliferation may be detrimental to osteogenesis. Other observations indicate that fibrous connective tissue/bone healing dynamics do not clearly demonstrate the demand for a completely cell-occlusive membrane design. The clinical probability of exposure in some cases, however, requires that the membrane have the potential for protecting the defect space from bacterial challenge in the event of membrane exposure. While there may be additional ways to provide this protection, the function of protection can be addressed, in part, by incorporating occlusive properties into the membrane structure.

Tissue integration appears to be an important criterion in the design of membranes for osseous regeneration in the oral cavity. In the event of membrane exposure to the oral cavity, tissue integration limits the migration of epithelium to keep pocketing, infection, and inflammation from interfering with the regenerative process. Membrane design must include an organized porous microstructure to encourage tissue integration for contact inhibition of the dentogingival epithelium as well as to create a mechanically stable site for optimum soft tissue and osseous healing. To determine the ideal membrane properties for tissue integration, thorough in vitro and in vivo tests appropriate to both the membrane material tested and the regenerative application treated are required.

The ability to create and maintain a given space with desired geometry adjacent to the parent bone surface is a critical requirement for successful GBR therapy. The spacemaking or resistance-to-collapse characteristics (stiffness) of a GBR membrane are important considerations in the choice of an appropriate membrane material. This is especially true for degradable materials, as they will lose mechanical strength during the degradation process. With currently available technology, stiffness of a GBR membrane must be balanced with conformability. Membranes with little or no resistance to collapse, or defects that have unfavorable membrane-supporting morphology, require the use of additional membrane supporting techniques.

Mechanical testing and physical characterization may predict how a specific membrane will behave when cut, shaped, secured in place, removed, or exposed to bacteria, and animal testing may indicate how the membrane performs when exposed to the oral environment of a particular animal model. However, clinical trials are necessary to establish the clinical performance value of a specific membrane design. Indeed, clinical trials with e-PTFE membranes were instrumental in developing surgical and postoperative management techniques.[3,4] Because clinical training and the quality of and compliance with medical care vary regionally and internationally, clinical trials in widely varied locations are necessary to establish the full range of clinical use requirements and efficacy. The balance of clinical manageability lies in designing a membrane for ease of use, performing clinical tests, then redesigning and incrementally improving the membrane for the best possible regenerative performance.

Experience has shown that for a GBR membrane to perform acceptably in the varied situations encountered in clinical practice, the membrane must incorporate a balanced set of features (form) that addresses specific requirements (function). Several of the requirements of an alveolar ridge GBR membrane are in conflict with one another (eg, tissue integration and bacterial occlusiveness), and the overall design must balance the needs of all requirements. It is also critical to take into account the specific advantages and disadvantages of a particular material. For example, a degradable material that will not require surgical removal must also provide structural integrity and spacemaking for a lengthy period. These considerations require sophisticated membrane design solutions.

It is hoped that the five GBR membrane design criteria discussed in this chapter will serve as a foundation and template for the design and testing of present and future GBR membrane materials. Many questions remain, particularly regarding the biologic mechanisms that operate during the complex hard and soft tissue healing events that are involved in alveolar ridge GBR. The resolution of these questions may identify additional functional requirements for GBR membranes. It will be the challenge of clinicians and material scientists to find innovative procedural and membrane design solutions to satisfy these requirements.

References

1. Dahlin C, Linde A, Gottlow J, Nyman S. Healing of bone defects by guided tissue regeneration. Plast Reconstr Surg 1988;81:672.

2. Dahlin C, Sennerby L, Lekholm U, Linde A, Nyman S. Generation of new bone around titanium implants using a membrane technique: An experimental study in rabbits. Int J Oral Maxillofac Implants 1989;4:19.

3. Buser D, Brägger U, Lang NP, Nyman S. Regeneration and enlargement of jaw bone using guided tissue regeneration. Clin Oral Impl Res 1990;1:22.

4. Becker W, Becker B. Guided tissue regeneration for implants placed into extraction sockets and for implant dehiscences: Surgical techniques and case reports. Int J Periodont Rest Dent 1990;10:377.

5. Williams DF. Biomaterials and biocompatibility: An introduction. In: Williams DF (ed). Fundamental Aspects of Biocompatibility, vol 1. Boca Raton, FL: CRC Press, 1981:1.

6. Coleman DL, King RN, Andrade JD. The foreign body reaction: A chronic inflammatory response. J Biomed Mater Res 1974;8:199.

7. Tripartite Biocompatibility Guidance for Medical Devices. General Purpose Memorandum #87-1 from the Director of the Office of Device Evaluation. FOI Document No. 104674. US Food and Drug Administration, Toxicology Subgroup of the Tripartite Sub-Committee on Medical Devices, 1986.

8. Boyce B. Physical characteristics of expanded polytetrafluoroethylene grafts. In: Stanley JC (ed). Biologic & Synthetic Vascular Prostheses. Philadelphia: Grune & Stratton, 1982:33.

9. Lewis DH. Controlled release of bioactive agents from lactide/glycolide polymers. In: Chasin M, Langer R (eds). Biodegradable Polymers as Drug Delivery Systems. New York: Marcel Dekker, 1990:1.

10. Böstman OM. Intense granulomatous inflammatory lesions associated with absorbable internal fixation devices made of polyglycolide in ankle fractures. Clin Orthop 1992;278:193.

11. Rae T. Cell biochemistry in relation to the inflammatory response to foreign materials. In: Williams DF (ed). Fundamental Aspects of Biocompatibility, vol 1. Boca Raton, FL: CRC Press, 1981:8.

12. Quteish D, Dolby AE. Immune responses to implanted human collagen graft in rats. J Periodont Res 1991;26:114.

13. Charnley J. Tissue reactions to polytetrafluoroethylene. Lancet 1963;2:1379.

14. Valentine JD, Reiman BEF, Beuttenmuller EA, Donovan MG. Light and electron microscopic evaluation of Proplast II TMJ disc implants. J Oral Maxillofac Surg 1989;47:689.

15. Somerman MJ, Sauk JJ, Foster RA, Dickerson K, Norris K, Argraves WS. Cell attachment activity of cementum: Bone sialoprotein II identified in cementum. J Periodont Res 1991;26:10.

16. Hurley LA, Stinchfield FE, Bassett CAL, Lyon WH. The role of soft tissues in osteogenesis. J Bone Joint Surg 1959;41a:1243.

17. Boyne PJ. Regeneration of alveolar bone beneath cellulose acetate filter implants. J Dent Res 1964;43:827.

18. Boyne PJ, Mikels TE. Restoration of alveolar ridges by intramandibular transposition osseous grafting. J Oral Surg 1968;26:569.

19. Boyne PJ. Restoration of osseous defects in maxillofacial casualties. J Am Dent Assoc 1969;78:767.

20. Karring T, Nyman S, Lindhe J. Healing following implantation of periodontitis-affected roots into bone tissue. J Clin Periodontol 1980;7:96.

21. Nyman S, Karring T, Lindhe J, Planten S. Healing following implantation of periodontitis-affected roots into gingival connective tissue. J Clin Periodontol 1980;7:394.

22. Karring T, Isidor F, Nyman S, Lindhe J. New attachment formation on teeth with a reduced but healthy periodontal ligament. J Clin Periodontol 1985;12:51.

23. Nyman S, Gottlow J, Karring T, Lindhe J. The regenerative potential of the periodontal ligament: An experimental study in the monkey. J Clin Periodontol 1982;9:257.

24. Nyman S, Lindhe J, Karring T, Rylander H. New attachment following surgical treatment of human periodontal disease. J Clin Periodontol 1982;9:290.

25. Melcher AH, Dreyer CJ. Protection of the blood clot in healing circumscribed bone defects. J Bone Joint Surg 1962;44b:424.

26. Aukhil I, Simpson DM, Schaberg TV. An experimental study of new attachment procedure in beagle dogs. J Periodont Res 1983;18:643.

27. Gottlow J, Nyman S, Karring T, Lindhe J. New attachment formation as the result of controlled tissue regeneration. J Clin Periodontol 1984;11:494.

28. Iglhaut J, Aukhil I, Simpson D, Johnston M, Koch G. Progenitor cell kinetics during guided tissue regeneration in experimental periodontal wounds. J Periodont Res 1988;23:107.

29. Magnusson I, Nyman S, Karring T, Egelberg J. Connective tissue attachment formation following exclusion of gingival connective tissue and epithelium during healing. J Periodont Res 1985;20:201.

30. Warrer K. Membranes for Periodontal Regeneration [thesis]. Aarhus, Denmark: Royal Dental College, 1990:34–48.

31. Ogiso B, Hughes FJ, Melcher AH, McCulloch CAG. Fibroblasts inhibit mineralized bone nodule formation by rat bone marrow stromal cells in vitro. J Cell Physiol 1991;146:442.

32. Murray G, Holden R, Roachlau W. Experimental and clinical study of new growth of bone in a cavity. Am J Surg 1957;93:385.

33. Farsø-Nielsen F, Karring T, Gogolewski S. Biodegradable guide for bone regeneration. Acta Orthop Scand 1992;63:66.

34. Linde A, Thoren C, Dahlin C, Sandberg E. Creation of new bone by an osteopromotive membrane technique. An experimental study in rats. J Oral Maxillofac Surg 1993;51:892.

35. Ilizarov GA. The tension-stress effect on the genesis and growth of tissues. Clin Orthop 1989;238:249.

36. Schenk RK. Biology of fracture repair. In: Brower BD, Jupiter JB, Levine AM, Trafton PG (eds). Skeletal Trauma. Philadelphia: Saunders,1992:31.

37. Warrer K, Gotfredsen K, Hjørting-Hansen E, Karring T. Guided tissue regeneration ensures osseointegration of dental implants placed into extraction sockets. An experimental study in monkeys. Clin Oral Impl Res 1991;2:166.

38. Winter G. Transcutaneous implants: Reactions of the skin-implant interface. J Biomed Mater Res Symp 1974;5:99.

39. Robinson WJ, Daly BDT Jr. Percutaneous leads for artificial hearts and other prosthetic devices. In: Szycher M, Robinson WJ (eds). Synthetic Biomedical Polymers. Lancaster, PA: Technomic, 1980.

40. Card SJ, Caffesse RG, Smith BA, Nasjleti CE. New attachment following the use of a resorbable membrane in the treatment of periodontitis in dogs. Int J Periodont Rest Dent 1989;9:59.

41. Warrer K, Karring T, Nyman S, Gogolewski S. Guided tissue regeneration using biodegradable membranes of polylactic acid or polyurethane. J Clin Periodontol 1992;19:633.

42. Caffesse RG, Smith BA, Castelli WA, Nasjleti CE. New attachment achieved by guided tissue regeneration in beagle dogs. J Periodontol 1988;59:589.

43. Kon S, Ruben MP, Bloom AA, Mardam-Bey W, Boffa J. Regeneration of periodontal ligament using resorbable and nonresorbable membranes: Clinical, histological and histometric study in dogs. Int J Periodont Rest Dent 1991;11:59.

44. Wolff J. Das Gesetz der Transformation der Knochen. Berlin: Hirschwalk, 1892.

45. Meachim G, Pedley RB. The tissue response at implant sites. In: Williams DF (ed). Fundamental Aspects of Biocompatibility, vol 1. Boca Raton, FL: CRC Press, 1981:6.

46. Whalen RL. Connective tissue response to movement at the prosthesis/tissue interface. In: Szycher M (ed). Biocompatible Polymers, Metals, and Composites. Lancaster, PA: Technomic, 1983:42.

47. Claffey N, Motsinger S, Ambruster J, Egelberg J. Placement of a porous membrane underneath the mucoperiosteal flap and its effect on periodontal wound healing in dogs. J Clin Periodontol 1989;16:12.

48. Haney JM, Nilvéus RE, McMillan PJ, Wikesjö UME. Periodontal repair in dogs: e-PTFE barrier membranes support wound stabilization and enhance bone regeneration. J Periodontol 1993;64:883.

49. Buser D, Dula K, Belser U, Hirt HP, Berthold H. Localized ridge augmentation using guided bone regeneration. I. Surgical procedure in the maxilla. Int J Periodont Rest Dent 1993;13:29.

50. Shanaman RH. The use of guided tissue regeneration to facilitate ideal prosthetic placement of implants. Int J Periodont Rest Dent 1992;12:257.

51. Mellonig JT, Triplett RG. Guided tissue regeneration and endosseous dental implants. Int J Periodont Rest Dent 1993;13:108.

52. Dahlin C, Gottlow J, Linde A, Nyman S. Healing of maxillary and mandibular bone defects using a membrane technique. An experimental study in monkeys. Scand J Plast Reconstr Surg 1990;24:13.

53. Seibert J, Nyman S. Localized ridge augmentation in dogs: A pilot study using membranes and hydroxyapatite. J Periodontol 1990;61:157.

54. Kohavi D, Pollack SR, Brighton G, Balkin B. Surgically modelled reduced ridge in the beagle dog. Clin Oral Impl Res 1991;2:145.

55. Pini Prato G, Tinti C, Vincenzi G, Magnani C, Cortellini P, Clauser C. Guided tissue regeneration versus mucogingival surgery in the treatment of human buccal gingival recession. J Periodontol 1992;63:919.

56. Hollinger J, Chaudhari A. Bone regeneration materials for the mandibular and craniofacial complex. Cell Mater 1992;2:143.

57. Becker W, Becker B. Guided tissue regeneration for implants placed into extraction sockets and for implant dehiscences: Surgical techniques and case reports. Int J Periodont Rest Dent 1990;10:377.

58. Schallhorn RG, McClain PK. Combined osseous grafting, root conditioning, and guided tissue regeneration. Int J Periodont Rest Dent 1988;8(4):9.

CHAPTER FIVE

Bone Promotion Around e-PTFE–Augmented Implants Placed in Immediate Extraction Sockets

William Becker
Burton E. Becker

The experimental and clinical investigations of Brånemark and coworkers[1–3] have provided periodontists, oral surgeons, and restorative dentists the biologic and clinical knowledge to predictably restore patients to proper function, comfort, and esthetics with implant-supported restorations. These restorations can be used to rehabilitate fully and partially edentulous patients as well as those requiring single-tooth replacements.[4–6] The traditional approach has been to remove hopeless teeth and wait from 4 months to 1 year to allow sufficient time for alveolar bone healing prior to implant placement. This chapter presents research data and clinical methods relating to implant placement in immediate extraction sockets.

The Problem

Surgeons, restorative dentists, and patients are uniquely aware of the problems associated with tooth extraction. Anatomically, there is resorption of the alveolar ridge in a buccolingual dimension as well as apicocoronally.[7] Over time, tissue compression from prosthetic appliances is responsible for loss of alveolar bone. In some patients the progressive loss of bone from poorly fitting dentures causes almost complete destruction of the alveolar bone, resulting in unstable dentures, pain during mastication, and eventual weight loss.

Biologic Studies

During the 1980s there was an explosion of research relating to periodontal regeneration.[8-11] The results of these studies indicated that if the periodontal ligament and surrounding alveolar bone could be isolated from gingival connective tissue and epithelium, it would be possible to regenerate the periodontium. Various types of materials have been used as barrier membranes; however, results after treatment with expanded polytetrafluoroethylene (e-PTFE, W.L. Gore, Flagstaff, AZ) have made these membranes the gold standard by which all others are compared. Over the past 12 years there have been numerous published papers attesting to the efficacy of barrier membranes for treatment of various periodontal defects.[12-14]

With the increased interest in and predictability of dental implants it was a natural evolution that membrane technology would be applied for promotion of bone adjacent to the implants. The original work of Dahlin et al[15] demonstrated that e-PTFE membranes can be used to promote bone around dehiscences adjacent to implants.

It has been demonstrated in an animal model that implants placed into fresh extraction sockets and augmented with barrier membranes have significant amounts of newly formed bone when compared with unaugmented controls.[16] Furthermore, at implant recovery the test sites had clinically significant increases in ridge width (Figs 5-1a to i). Histologic evaluation of the test specimens demonstrated new bone formation in contact with the titanium implant surface and almost 100% bone coverage of the previously exposed threads. Control specimens demonstrated very little new bone formation over the previously exposed threads. Similar results have been reported by other investigators.[17]

Lekholm and coworkers[18] performed an experimental study to determine the effect of premature membrane removal on bone formation around dental implants. Sites in which the membranes were retained for the entire healing interval had the greatest clinical increases in bone formation (5.2 mm). Sites in which only the membranes were removed had an average of 2.0 mm of new bone. Sites in which the membranes and underlying granulation tissue were removed had an average of 1.0 mm of bone regeneration. Histologic evaluation of the granulation tissue biopsy specimens demonstrated minimal signs of inflammation, with the occasional presence of bone spicules at the implant coronal aspect. Histologic evaluation of ground sections of the bone and implant specimens verified the clinical findings. Sites in which the membranes were retained had 100% new bone formation over the previously exposed threads. In most sections, new bone had

Barrier membranes promote bone growth around implants placed in immediate extraction sockets in dogs.
Figs 5-1a to i

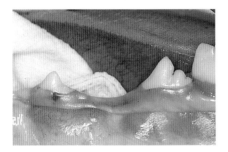

5-1a

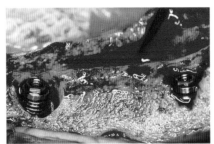

5-1b

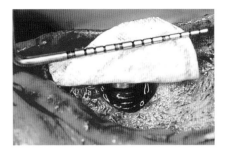

5-1c

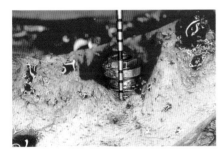

5-1d

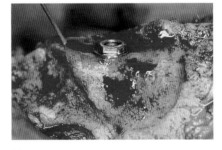

5-1e

Fig 5-1a   Canine mandibular molars prior to extraction.

Fig 5-1b   Molars have been removed and the openings to the extraction sockets have been enlarged. Standard Nobelpharma 10-mm implants have been inserted into the extraction sockets.

Fig 5-1c   An e-PTFE barrier membrane has been fixed to the test implant with the cover screw. The distal implant is the control.

Fig 5-1d   Control site at 12-week retrieval period. Note thread exposure and incomplete coverage of the threads.

Fig 5-1e   Test site at 12 weeks. Note total coverage of previously exposed threads and increase in ridge width.

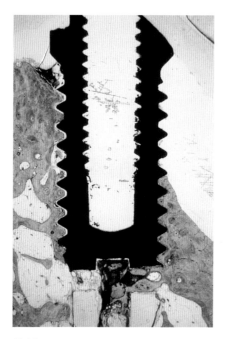

5-1f

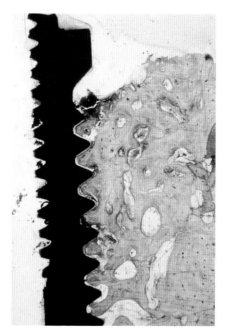

5-1g

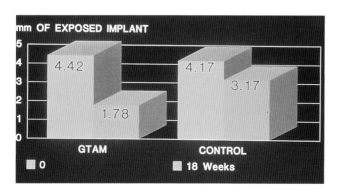

5-1h

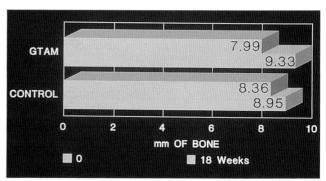

5-1i

Fig 5-1f Histologic section of control site. Note five exposed threads.

Fig 5-1g Histologic section of test site. Note complete bone-to-implant coverage of implant threads and enlarged bone width.

Fig 5-1h Mean midbuccal changes in bone height for test and control sites.

Fig 5-1i Mean changes in bone width for test and control sites. (Reprinted with permission from Becker et al.[16])

grown over the top of the implants. In contrast, specimens in which the membranes were removed alone or with underlying tissue had significantly less new bone with a greater number of threads exposed.

These results verify the clinical findings of Simeon et al[19] and have clinical ramifications. To promote maximum bone formation around implants that have been augmented with barrier membranes, it is imperative that the material remain in place, immobilized and covered by the flap mucosa for the entire healing period.

Rationale for Immediate Implant Placement

Lazzara[20] first discussed the concept of placing implants into immediate extraction sockets and augmenting these sites with e-PTFE barrier membranes. Since his original paper, numerous authors have published case histories and clinical results relating to immediate implant placement with barrier membranes. The majority of these reports relate to one- or two-tooth implant replacements.[21]

The principal reason for using this procedure is to preserve the alveolar ridge width and height, thereby preserving the maximum amount of bone for implant placement. Secondary reasons are the potential decreased restorative interval between tooth removal and implant restoration and the psychological ramifications for patients who have a phobia about losing their teeth.

Dental conditions that might be good indications for immediate implant placement are root fractures, failed endodontic therapy, and advanced periodontal disease. Teeth with unrestorable carious lesions or poor crown-to-root ratios might also be good candidates for immediate implant placement.

Clinical Procedures

Diagnosis and Treatment Planning

Proper diagnosis and treatment planning are critical to successful treatment outcome. This is especially true for immediate implant placement in the maxillary anterior region of the mouth. Factors that must be taken into consideration are lip and smile line, gingival thickness, presence or absence of periodontal disease adjacent to the tooth to be removed, and bone quality and quantity. The Lekholm and Zarb[22] method for classifying bone quality and quantity has recently been modified to include jawbone anatomy with teeth present.[23]

Changes in Bone Quality with Teeth Present
(Modification of Lekholm and Zarb Classification[22])

A1. No attachment loss, endodontic involvement (root fracture, possible periapical pathosis)

B1. Loss of one third of periodontal attachment

C1. Loss of one half of periodontal attachment

D1. Loss of three fourths of periodontal attachment

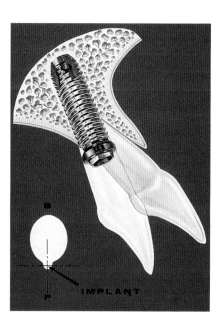

Fig 5-2 Migration of a tooth with advanced periodontal disease. The implant must be placed in the palatal aspect of the socket; placement of the implant in the tooth position will give an unfavorable angulation to the implant. B = buccal; P = palatal. (Drawing courtesy of D. Brunel.)

To achieve implant stability there should be a minimum of 3 to 5 mm of bone apical to the root apex. The basic radiographic examination should consist of periapical and panoramic radiographs. Evaluation of the radiographs should demonstrate sufficient bone for implant placement without traumatizing the neurovascular bundle, maxillary sinus, or adjacent teeth.

An understanding of tooth anatomy and position is necessary for successful implant placement. Maxillary anterior teeth with advanced periodontal diseases migrate in a labial direction (Fig 5-2). A diagnostic waxup must be used during the treatment planning phase to visualize the teeth in their original positions. The surgical implant stent is then fabricated and used during surgery. Once the teeth have been removed and the stent has been placed in proper position, the surgeon will note that the implants will be placed in the most palatal aspect of the extraction sockets. If the implants were to be placed in the diseased or flared positions, they would be too far labially, culminating in a restorative and esthetic disaster.

Surgical Procedures

To reduce the incidence of postoperative infection, patients should be placed on an appropriate antibiotic 2 hours prior to surgery.[24] Furthermore, implants must not be placed into an area of suppuration. Immediate implant placement requires attention to detail. For practical purposes, the surgical steps are divided into six phases: flap design, extraction, site preparation, implant placement, implant augmentation, and flap closure.

Flap Design

Proper flap design is one of the most critical steps in the procedure.[23] Two flap designs are described in this chapter: flaps used when teeth are adjacent to the tooth being extracted (Figs 5-3a to d) and those used when the tooth to be replaced is adjacent to an edentulous ridge (Figs 5-4a to c).[23] Both types of flaps require extension of the anterior aspect of the flap one tooth anterior to the tooth to be extracted. A reversed C-shaped vertical incision is extended past the mucogingival junction. Full-thickness mucoperiosteal flaps are reflected buccally to expose the vestibular aspect of the alveolar bone and palatally to fully visualize the alveolar ridge. In the mandibular arch, the mental nerve is exposed to prevent accidental nerve encroachment.

Tooth Extraction

Atraumatic extraction of the tooth to be replaced requires patience and a gentle technique. To preserve the entire buccal plate, small elevators are used with primarily mesiodistal luxation. This step must be performed slowly and usually requires several minutes to accomplish. The extraction forceps are not applied until the tooth is extremely mobile. Failure to follow these steps can lead to root fracture or fracture of the surrounding bony plate, both of which may require cancellation of the procedure.

Site Preparation

Thorough debridement of the extraction socket can be accomplished with a combination of small periodontal files and curettes. All visible granulation tissue must be extirpated from the socket. Once the socket has been thoroughly debrided it must be gently flushed with sterile saline. To avoid contamination of the implant surgical instruments, the debridement instruments are removed from the surgical field.

Once the tooth has been removed, the surgeon must choose the most appropriate site for implant placement. The preliminary waxup and stent will be of value, but the final decision is made after careful inspection of the alveolar socket and surrounding bone. In the maxillary incisors and premolar regions, the implant will usually be placed in the palatal aspect of the socket. In the maxillary molars, the implant can be placed in the interradicular bone. In some instances, the palatal root is also a suitable site for

Flap design procedure:
Teeth adjacent to tooth being extracted.

Figs 5-3a to d

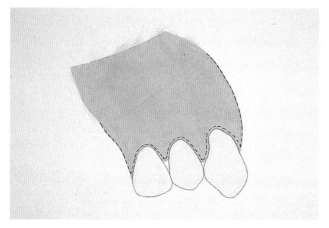

5-3a

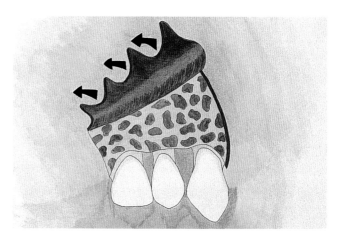

5-3b

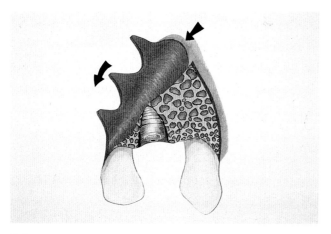

5-3c

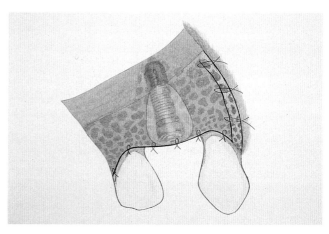

5-3d

Fig 5-3a   Flap design for removal of a maxillary premolar adjacent to two noninvolved teeth.

Fig 5-3b   Full-thickness flaps are reflected, exposing the underlying bone.

Fig 5-3c   Premolar is removed. A small buccal dehiscence is present.

Fig 5-3d   Implant is placed and augmented with an e-PTFE barrier. A pedicle flap from the canine is rotated distally, providing total coverage of the augmented implant. The vertical incision is sutured, leaving a small island of bone exposed. (Figs 5-3a, c, and d reprinted with permission from Becker et al.[23])

Flap design and procedure:
Edentulous ridge adjacent to tooth being extracted.
Figs 5-4a to c

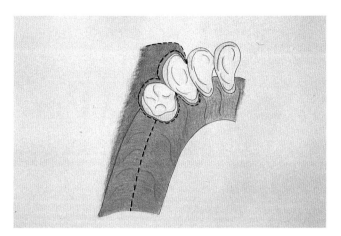

5-4a

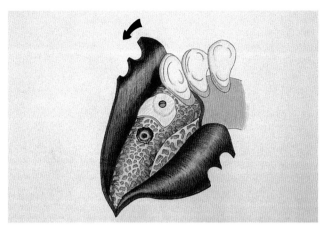

5-4b

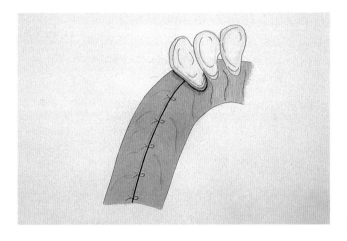

5-4c

Fig 5-4a Flap design for removal of a mandibular premolar adjacent to edentulous ridge.

Fig 5-4b Premolar is removed, and implant is placed and augmented with an e-PTFE membrane.

Fig 5-4c Pedicle flap is rotated from the canine distally, providing complete coverage of the augmented implant. The flaps are sutured with horizontal and interrupted sutures. (Figs 5-4a to c reprinted with permission from Becker et al.[23])

implant placement. In the mandibular molars, the interradicular bone and mesial and distal sockets can be used as sites for implant placement. If there is adequate space, implants can be placed in the mesial and distal sockets; however, it has been our experience that one implant is sufficient to replace a mandibular molar.

Implant Placement

Prior to site preparation, the surgical stent is positioned and stabilized. A round bur is used to prepare an occlusal-apical notch at the palatal aspect of the extraction socket. This groove will serve as a guide for the initial drilling and will help prevent the drill from moving from the ideal preparation site. Standard drilling procedures are used, dependent on the implant system being used. Prior to implant insertion, the implant site must be carefully measured. The head of the implant must be at or slightly inferior to the alveolar crest. In the mandible, if the measurement indicates that the site was not prepared deep enough, and if further deepening will encroach on the mandibular canal, the implant must be downsized. If a titanium screw-type implant is used, a countersink preparation is made. The decision to tap is determined by the bone quality. In the posterior maxilla, standard 3.75-mm implants are inserted without tapping. In the mandible, the coronal one third of the site may be tapped. Standard or self-tapping implants are then inserted under a continuous stream of chilled sterile saline. Once the implant has been placed, the surgeon must decide whether the site should be augmented.

Implant-Bone Augmentation Considerations

The depth and width of the residual defect surrounding the implant are the most relevant factors for determining whether to augment the implant site. The clinician must always assess the problem and consider the risk-to-benefit relationship prior to initiating any procedure. Narrow, shallow defects less than 3 mm probably do not need to be augmented. If the defect is greater than 3 mm and there are several threads exposed, augmentation should be considered. The important question to answer is: *Will the newly formed bone significantly add to the load-bearing capabilities of the implant?* If the answer is *yes*, the site must be augmented.

The purpose of placing an e-PTFE barrier membrane over the implant is to maintain the space surrounding the implant. The blood clot filling the space will become organized with a callus that will eventually become organized into newly formed bone. The surgeon has several barriers from which to choose. The membrane is placed over the implanted site. There must be 1 to 2 mm of space between the lateral borders of the membrane and the adjacent teeth. If the membrane is in contact with adjacent teeth, it can be trimmed. The membrane can be fixed to the implant with the cover screw, or draped over the implant and tucked under the flap margins.

Flap Closure

Flap closure is one of the most important aspects of the procedure. A pedicle flap from the anterior flap extension is dissected from the underlying periosteum and rotated distally. Flap rotation should place minimal tension on the pedicle. Once the pedicle has been placed over the augmented implant, horizontal mattress sutures are used to coapt the flap margins. This usually requires the placement of two horizontal mattress sutures. Upon completion of flap closure, the wound must be inspected for material exposure. If the membrane is not completely covered by the mucosal flap, it should be resutured. Patients are instructed to apply ice and gentle pressure to the surgical site for 24 hours. The sutures are removed in 1 week and the wound is inspected for closure. Patients are seen bimonthly for 2 months. In most instances, the material remains covered and is not removed until the abutment connection. Figures 5-5a to p show the step-by-step procedure for placing a single implant into an extraction socket with an e-PTFE barrier membrane.

Material Exposure

In the event that the material becomes exposed during the first 6 to 8 weeks after implant placement, the wound can be cleansed with daily applications of 0.12% chlorhexidine. After 8 weeks, the area is anesthetized and a partial-thickness flap is made adjacent to the augmented site. The barrier is gently removed, and the flap margins are sutured. If the material was retained with a cover screw, a new, sterile cover screw should be secured to the implant. The granulation tissue beneath the membrane must not be disturbed. The sutures are removed in 1 week and the implant is left undisturbed until the abutment connection.

Barrier Membrane Removal at Abutment Connection

At the abutment connection, a mucosal flap is made over the augmented implant. The margins of the material are delineated, and the barrier is dissected free of the underlying bone. The wound must be carefully inspected to assure that all remnants of material have been completely removed. The bone surrounding the implant is then inspected and appropriate healing abutments are fixed to the implant. Restoration of the implant is completed in the normal manner.

Placement of an implant in an immediate extraction socket of a mandibular right premolar.

Figs 5-5a to p

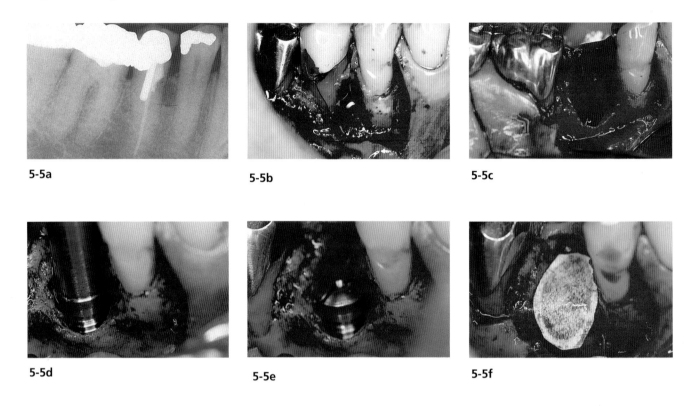

5-5a

5-5b

5-5c

5-5d

5-5e

5-5f

Fig 5-5a   Periapical radiograph demonstrating inadequate endodontic treatment and mesial horizontal bone loss of the premolar.

Fig 5-5b   Buccal full-thickness flap is reflected, revealing a vertical root fracture of the mandibular second premolar.

Fig 5-5c   Premolar is removed, and site is thoroughly debrided and prepared with appropriate drills. The site has an occlusal countersink and was tapped.

Fig 5-5d   Standard 13-mm implant (Nobelpharma) is placed.

Fig 5-5e   Implant cover screw is fixed to the implant. Three threads are exposed and there is a 3-mm mesiodistal gap between the implant and surrounding bone.

Fig 5-5f   Augmentation material (Gore-Tex, W.L. Gore) is trimmed to avoid contact with adjacent teeth and placed over the implant.

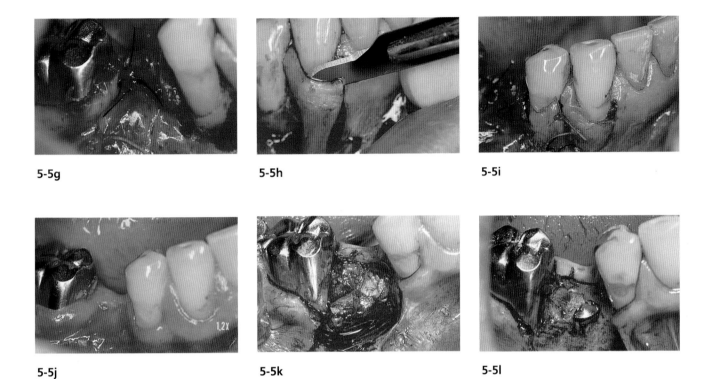

5-5g

5-5h

5-5i

5-5j

5-5k

5-5l

Fig 5-5g   Pedicle flap is rotated distally from the first premolar and sutured over the augmented implant.

Fig 5-5h   Partial-thickness pedicle flap is dissected from the facial aspect of the canine.

Fig 5-5i   Pedicle graft from the canine is sutured in place over the facial aspect of the first premolar.

Fig 5-5j   Surgical site 11 months postoperatively. One suture is retained.

Fig 5-5k   Mucosal flap is reflected, exposing the underlying barrier membrane. The membrane is completely dissected free from the underlying bone.

Fig 5-5l   Note bone covering one half of implant cover screw. This bone was removed with small chisels, a standard nonrotating abutment was placed onto the implant hex head.

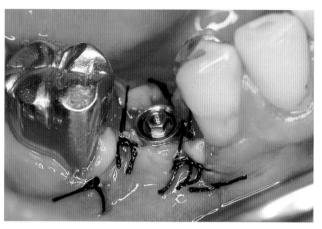

5-5m

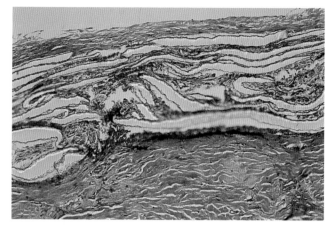

5-5n

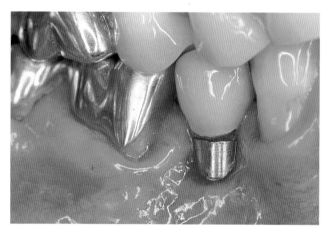

5-5o

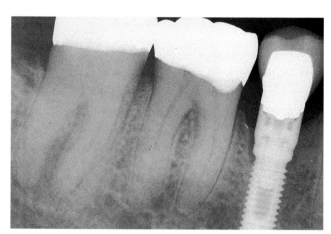

5-5p

Fig 5-5m Flap is apically positioned on the facial aspect of the abutment cylinder.

Fig 5-5n Histologic view of retrieved barrier. Note healthy connective tissue, blood vessels, and absence of inflammatory cells above and below the membrane.

Fig 5-5o Single-tooth restoration is placed on the implant.

Fig 5-5p Periapical radiograph taken 3.5 years after loading. There is crestal bone loss to the first thread.

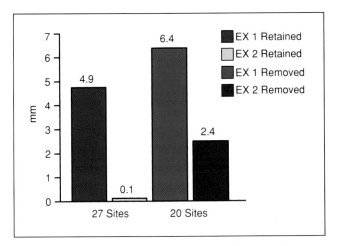

Fig 5-6 Changes in bone height for membranes retained and membranes that became exposed and were removed early.[23]

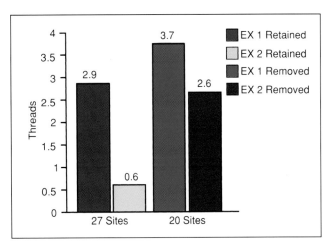

Fig 5-7 Changes in thread exposure for membrane-retained sites and sites in which the membranes were removed early.[23]

Results of a Multicenter Study

Short-term evaluations of implants augmented with e-PTFE barrier membranes have been encouraging, as shown in a recently published prospective multicenter study.[23] The short-term implant survival rate is 93.9% and the amount of new bone surrounding the implants has been impressive (4.6 mm for membrane-retained sites). Of the 49 implants evaluated, 3 were lost prior to the abutment connection (Figs 5-6 and 5-7).[23]

Important clinical information was obtained from the patients in whom the implants failed. These implants were placed in patients who became fully edentulous with the loss of their remaining teeth. Their provisional dentures were inadequately relined, and the patients were not frequently monitored. The dentures perforated the mucosa, and the underlying membranes became contaminated by bacteria and subsequently became infected. Clinicians should use caution when using barriers in patients who will wear complete dentures as provisional restorations. Furthermore, multiple membranes may embarrass the blood supply to the flap, making the flap susceptible to dehiscence and material exposure.

Alloplasts, Allografts, and Autologous Grafts Beneath Barrier Membranes

There have been numerous reports attesting to the bone-promoting qualities of various types of implant augmentation materials, yet there are very few animal or prospective clinical studies evaluating these materials. In general, these materials are used as space maintainers to keep the barriers from collapsing against the implants. In reality, they may displace the blood clot and minimize the space against the implant and may actually limit the amount of potential new bone formation. Animal studies that evaluated alloplastic materials produced inconsistent results with minimal amounts of new bone.[25] These materials are not osteoinductive and have not been proven to increase the loading capabilities of the implants.

Demineralized freeze-dried cortical bone allografts have been used extensively for treatment of periodontal defects with and without barrier membranes.[26–28] The allografts are thought to contain bone morphogenetic proteins (BMPs).[29] However, commercial bone banks do not verify the presence of BMPs in the material. To date, there are no convincing data that would indicate that this type of graft has any osteoinductive potential when used to augment dental implants. Furthermore, there is no evidence that allografts add to the loading capability of the implant. To the contrary, there is recent experimental evidence that the particles of calcified allograft material may actually impede bone formation.[30]

In a recently reported animal experimental study,[31] human bone (xenografts), insulin I, and platelet-derived growth factors were used beneath e-PTFE membranes and compared with membranes alone for bone-promoting qualities. Sites that received the bone grafts did not demonstrate any evidence of rejection and had the greatest variability in terms of new bone formation. In the majority of sites, this material gave the poorest clinical and histologic results. The greatest amount of new bone was found at sites where growth factors were used and at sites that were only augmented with membranes. Results of these experimental studies suggest that allograft material in small quantities may not be as osteoinductive as was originally suggested and that its use may interject an unknown variable into the healing sequence.

Autologous bone grafting has an extensive history of use in orthopedic surgery.[32,33] In studies comparing autografts and allografts it is concluded that autologous bone is the best type of graft to use for orthopedic purposes.[32,33] There are no studies which confirm that autologous grafts actually promote bone adjacent to the implant; however, if a material is needed to create or maintain a space beneath a barrier, autogenous bone should be the graft material of choice. Small particles of autogenous bone can be readily harvested from the lateral bone margins of the implant site, from the maxillary tuberosity, or from retromolar areas. While the procurement of bone from sites away from the main surgical field creates a second surgical incision, the use of autologous bone has a far greater potential for maintaining cell viability compared with allografts.

References

1. Adell R, Lekholm U, Rockler B, Brånemark P-I. A 15-year study of osseointegrated implants in the treatment of the edentulous jaw. Int J Oral Surg 1981; 10:387.

2. Albrektsson T, Dahl E, Enbom L, Engevall S, Engquist B, Eriksson AR, et al. Osseointegrated oral implants. A Swedish multicenter study of 8139 consecutively inserted Nobelpharma implants. J Periodontol 1988;59:287.

3. Adell R, Eriksson B, Lekholm U, Brånemark P-I, Jemt T. A long-term follow-up study of osseointegrated implants in the treatment of the totally edentulous jaw. Int J Oral Maxillofac Implants 1990;5:347.

4. van Steenberghe D, Quirynen M, Calberson L, Demanet M. A prospective evaluation of the fate of 697 consecutive intraoral fixtures ad modem Brånemark in the rehabilitation of edentulism. J Head Neck Pathol 1987;6:53.

5. Jemt T, Lekholm U, Grondahl K. A 3-year followup study of early single implant restorations ad modum Brånemark. Int J Periodont Rest Dent 1990; 10:341.

6. van Steenberghe D, Lekholm U, Folmer T, Henry P, Herrmann I, Higuchi K, et al. The applicability of osseointegrated oral implants in the rehabilitation of partial edentulism. A prospective multicenter study of 558 fixtures. Int J Oral Maxillofac Implants 1990;5:272.

7. Atwood DA. Postextraction changes in the adult mandible as illustrated by microradiographs of mid-sagital sections and serial cephalometric roentgenographs. J Prosthet Dent 1963;13:810.

8. Nyman S, Lindhe J, Karring T, Rylander H. New attachment following surgical treatment of human periodontal disease. J Clin Periodontol 1982;9:290.

9. Gottlow J, Nyman S, Karring T, Lindhe J. New attachment formation as a result of controlled tissue regeneration. J Clin Periodontol 1984;11:494.

10. Gottlow J, Nyman S, Lindhe J, Karring T, Wennstrom J. New attachment formation in the human periodontium by guided tissue regeneration: Case reports. J Clin Periodontol 1986;13:604.

11. Becker W, Becker BE, Berg L, Prichard J, Caffesse R, Rosenberg E, et al. Root isolation for new attachment procedures: A surgical and suturing method: Three case reports. J Periodontol 1987;58:819.

12. Becker W, Becker BE, Berg L, Prichard J, Caffesse R, Rosenberg E. New attachment after treatment with root isolation procedures: Report for treated Class III and Class II furcations and vertical osseous defects. Int J Periodont Rest Dent 1988;8(3):9.

13. Schallhorn R, McClain P. Combined osseous composite grafting, root conditioning and guided tissue regeneration. Int J Periodont Rest Dent 1988;8(4):9.

14. Caffesse R, Smith BA, Duff B, Morrison EC, Merrill D, Becker W. Class II furcations treated by guided tissue regeneration in humans: Case reports. J Periodontol 1990;8:510.

15. Dahlin C, Sennerby L, Lekholm U, Linde A, Nyman S. Generation of new bone around titanium implants: An experimental study in rabbits. Int J Oral Maxillofac Implants 1989;4:19.

16. Becker W, Becker BE, Handelsman M, Ochsenbein C, Albrektsson T. Guided tissue regeneration for implants placed into extraction sockets: A study in dogs. J Periodontol 1991;62:703.

17. Caudill RF, Meffert RM. Histologic analysis of the osseointegration of endosseous implants in simulated extraction sockets with and without e-PTFE barriers. Int J Periodont Rest Dent 1991;11:207.

18. Lekholm U, Becker W, Dahlin C, Becker BE, Donath K, Morrison E. The role of early vs late removal of GTAM-membranes on bone formation around oral implants placed in immediate extraction sockets: An experimental study in dogs. Clin Oral Impl Res 1993;4:121–129.

19. Simion M, Baldoni J, Zaffe D. Rigenerazione guidata dei tessuti in osteointegrazione: Site post-extrattive. Rivistas Italiana di Osteointsegrazione 1991;1:40.

20. Lazzara R. Immediate implant placement into extraction sites: Surgical and restorative advantages. Int J Periodont Rest Dent 1989;9:333.

21. Becker W, Becker BE. Guided tissue regeneration for implants placed into extraction sockets and for implant dehiscences: Surgical techniques and case reports. Int J Periodont Rest Dent 1990;10:377.

22. Lekholm U, Zarb GA. Patient selection and preparation. In: Brånemark P-I, Albrektsson T, Zarb GA (eds). Tissue-Integrated Prostheses: Osseointegration in Clinical Dentistry. Chicago: Quintessence, 1985:199.

23. Becker W, Dahlin C, Becker BE, Lekholm U, van Steenberghe D, Higuchi K, Kultje C. The use of e-PTFE barrier membranes for bone promotion around titanium implants placed into extraction sockets: A prospective multicenter study. Int J Oral Maxillofac Implants 1994;9:31–40.

24. Classen DC, Scott E, Stanley L, Pestotnik SL, et al. The timing of prophylactic administration of antibiotics and the risk of surgical-wound infection. New Engl J Med 1992;326:281.

25. Wachtel HC, Langford A, Bernimoulin JP, Reichart P. Guided bone regeneration next to osseointegrated implants in humans. Int J Oral Maxillofac Implants 1991;6:127.

26. Mellonig J, Bowers G, Bright R. Clinical evaluation of freeze dried allograft in periodontal osseous defects. J Periodontol 1976;47:125.

27. Quintero G, Mellonig J, Gambil V. A six month clinical evaluation of decalcified freeze dried bone allograft in human periodontal defects. J Periodontol 1982;53:726.

28. Anderegg CR, Martin S, Gray J, Mellonig J. Clinical evaluation of the use of decalcified freeze dried bone allograft with guided tissue regeneration in the treatment of molar furcation invasions. J Periodontol 1991;62:264.

29. Urist MR, Huo YK, Brownell AG, Gher M. Purification of bovine bone morphogenetic protein by hydroxyapatite chromatography. Proc Natl Acad Sci 1984;81:371.

30. Sampatha R, Werther JR, Hauschka PV. Accelerated endochrondral osteoinduction in the absence of bone matrix particles in a rat model system. J Oral Maxillofac Surg 1992;50:140.

31. Becker W, Lynch S, Lekholm U, Becker BE, et al. A comparison of e-PTFE membranes alone or in combination with platelet-derived growth factors and insulin-like growth factor-I or demineralized freeze-dried bone in promoting bone formation around immediate extraction socket implants. J Periodontol 1992;63:929.

32. Goldberg VM, Stevenson S. Natural history of autografts and allografts. Clin Orthop Rel Res 1987;225:7.

33. Friedlander GE. Current concepts review. Bone grafts: The basic science rationale for clinical applications. J Bone Joint Surg 1987;69:786.

CHAPTER SIX

Guided Bone Regeneration in Dehiscence Defects and Delayed Extraction Sockets

Sascha A. Jovanovic
Daniel Buser

At the time of implant placement, anatomic bone deficiencies will result in exposed implant surfaces, reduced bone-to-implant contact, and, as a consequence, compromised results varying from early implant failures to late peri-implant infections.[1] Anatomic indications of membrane utilization to improve these clinical entities for the regeneration of new bone over exposed implant surfaces can be divided into three main groups:

Anatomic Indications for Membrane Use in Implant Sites

Group I. Sites with an anatomic insufficiency of crest width resulting in an exposed implant surface

Group II. Sites in which the prosthetically guided placement of an implant results in exposure of the buccal implant surface (this can include the intentional perforation of the buccal surface)

Group III. Sites where voids exist between the implant and the bone when an implant is placed into an extraction socket

Implant surface exposures in sites such as dehiscence defects, fenestration defects, and/or extraction sockets can be found in these three groups. Clinical testing of the membrane technique in these indications has shown encouraging results.[2–10]

Experimental and clinical research of membrane therapy has led to an increase in indications for implant placement in sites previously thought to be unsuitable (Fig 6-1a). However, membrane therapy should not be applied beyond the biologic tolerance. To improve the predictability of new bone formation over exposed implant surfaces, a superficial dehiscence-type defect within the alveolar crest is preferred over an implant positioned outside the alveolar housing. This assumption is based on the hypothesis that bone formation is primarily determined by the degree of vascularization taking place from the apical and lateral bone margins. In addition, cells originating from the bone tissue should not be expected to migrate over extreme distances.[11]

At the present time, indications for membrane placement to ensure a highly predictable outcome should therefore be restricted to moderate defects such as superficial dehiscence defects, fenestration defects, and extraction sockets within the alveolar housing. If a larger defect is present, the addition of a bone graft is recommended.

Preoperative diagnosis is necessary to predict these compromised sites and to evaluate presurgically whether they are suitable for simultaneous placement of an implant and a barrier membrane. Appropriate diagnostic procedures include intraoral bone mapping and radiographic techniques.[12] Furthermore, the cross-sectional views of the jawbone demonstrated by a conventional tomogram (Fig 6-1b) or a CT scan can be very helpful.[13,14] The decision whether a simultaneous approach can be utilized should be based on the necessity of primary stability of the implant as well as the size and morphology of the peri-implant bone defect.[6,9,15]

Ideal Implant Placement

After the extraction of natural teeth, the greatest reduction of the alveolar bone occurs in the first 6 months to 2 years.[16] This ridge resorption will determine the position and angulation of the implant.[17] For the implant to be engaged in the optimum width of bone, it is often necessary that the implant be tipped buccally. This angulation can result in an emergence of the screw-access hole through the buccal aspect of the implant restoration, and in an implant that is not positioned axially to occlusal forces. Esthetic and functional problems can result.

In contrast, if the implant is placed in an optimal position for an esthetic and functional restoration, a dehiscence or fenestration defect can be expected. This exposed implant surface can be treated by utilizing the guided bone regeneration (GBR) technique, either in conjunction with implant placement **(simultaneous approach)** or as a ridge augmentation procedure before implant placement **(staged approach)**.[15,18,19] Clinicians should realize that implants placed in positions that create large dehiscence or fenestration defects have an increased risk of failure should the regenerative procedure fail or an infection occur. Thus, as in every surgical procedure, diagnosis and careful risk/benefit evaluation must be employed.

Guided Bone Regeneration in Dehiscence Defects

Incision Technique and Flap Design

To ensure an optimal outcome of a membrane-assisted treatment, an undisturbed submerged healing of the membrane is essential. This has been demonstrated in clinical[6,7,18] as well as experimental studies.[20-22] Exposed membranes have an increased risk of infection and can result in bone loss rather than bone formation.[6,18] Therefore, a surgical protocol that allows primary soft tissue healing should be followed.[9,15,23] To decrease the overall risk of infection when using an alloplastic material, presurgical antimicrobial therapy, including preoperative antibiotic coverage and intraoral rinsing with chlorhexidine (0.12%), is performed.

A split- to full-thickness remote flap design is planned, and an incision is made 5 mm toward the palatal side of the maxillary crest, or 4 mm below the buccal mucogingival junction of the mandibular crest (Figs 6-1c and d). The initial incision is kept shallow but perpendicular to the bone. This is followed by a supraperiosteal preparation toward the crest of the ridge. The periosteum is incised as close as possible to the midcrest. Vertical releasing incisions enhance flap mobility, and are placed at least one tooth width away from the anticipated margin of the membrane.

The mucoperiosteal flaps are carefully elevated (Fig 6-1e) to preserve all of the periosteum. They are reflected buccally in the case of a palatal incision, or lingually in the case of an incision below the buccal mucogingival junction. The opposite wound margins are elevated, creating a space in which the membrane can be tucked. To minimize trauma to the periosteum by surgical retractors, the flap is held away by retraction sutures.

Bone Preparation

The local bone bed surrounding the implant recipient site is the source of the cells that contribute to the bone formation response and the source of nutrition to these cells through vascular formation.[24] Because of the critical role the local tissue bed plays in any regenerative procedure, it should be handled with care; preparation should facilitate the activation of osteoprogenitor cells.

After meticulous elevation of the flap with an appropriate tissue elevator, the bone surface is examined for the presence of pathologic changes. If present, this tissue is carefully and thoroughly removed with a surgical curette. In addition, local bone surfaces should be prepared to present the greatest possible surface area of healthy vascular bone to the membrane site, and all soft tissue remnants should be removed from the bone surface.[18,23] The preparation of cortical bone is best performed with a surgical curette or round burs. Potential sources of local osteogenic cells are found particularly in bone and bone marrow.[25,26] Therefore, the perforation of the cortical bone to open the marrow space enables the access of osteoprogenitor and angiogenic cells to the bone defect. The blood clot will provide the matrix for an appropriate healing response.[27] Various growth factors are released by platelets and other local cells. These elements are part of the normal healing process for bone formation.

Implant and Membrane Placement

An appropriate implant site—one that combines the optimal bone bed with an appropriate implant position from a prosthetic point of view—is chosen (Figs 6-1f to h). Implant dehiscence outside the alveolar housing should be kept moderate in size to facilitate complete regeneration with new bone and sufficient primary stability of the implant.[10] If an implant dehiscence is protruding beyond the alveolar housing, or is more than 5 mm in length, autogenous bone grafts should be used to fill the created space between the implant and the overlying membrane (Figs 6-1i and j). This will aid in space maintenance of the membrane and in bone formation.[5,9]

The membrane barrier is trimmed with scissors so that the stiffer inner portion covers the defect, and, thus, an appropriate space between the implant and the membrane is created. The flexible outer portion of the membrane overlaps the periphery of the bone defect by approximately 3 to 5 mm. Sharp corners of the material are rounded to prevent flap perforation by the membrane and to allow close adaptation of the membrane to the surrounding bone surface to avoid the ingrowth of gingival connective tissue cells. The importance of the development of a protected space for consistent new bone formation has also been demonstrated in other experimental studies without membranes.[28,29]

Fixation of the membrane barrier is preferred, since movements of the membrane can influence the outcome of the bone healing response. Membrane movement can result in loss of the close adaptation of the membrane to the bone surface, and will thus facilitate the ingrowth of soft tissue cells. In addition, micromovement may promote the formation of fibrous tissue, as has been demonstrated for dental implants.[30] To stabilize and immobilize the membrane, cover screws or/and fixation screws can be used (Fig 6-1k). Clinical experience has clearly demonstrated that the use of membrane-fixation devices has greatly improved the predictability of the GBR technique.[4,6,9,15,18] After fixation, the membrane is adapted on the opposite aspect of the alveolar ridge by placing the membrane underneath the palatal/lingual mucoperiosteal flap. For ideal bone healing, three goals must be achieved through membrane placement: *(1)* creation of a protected space in the defect area, *(2)* adaptation of the membrane to the surrounding bone surface, and *(3)* immobilization of the membrane.

Wound Closure and Postoperative Treatment

During flap closure, all tension should be minimized to avoid exposure of the membrane and to avoid excessive pressure on the membrane resulting in space reduction. This can be achieved by incising the periosteum at the base of the buccal flap. The lingual flap is often too thin to allow an incision of the periosteum. In these cases, larger mucoperiosteal elevation will aid in tension-free adaptation of the wound margin.

Primary wound closure is obtained by mattress and interrupted sutures. The mattress sutures including the periosteal layer provide stabilization of the wound (Fig 6-1l). In addition, these sutures sustain the postoperative flap tension created by the swelling within the wound in the first 3 days following surgery. The interrupted sutures provide close adaptation of the wound margins to facilitate rapid primary healing (Fig 6-1m).

Healing Period and Membrane Removal

An important factor for the GBR technique is the length of the healing period. At present, the minimum time to regenerate peri-implant defects covered with barrier membranes is unknown, and is probably patient and site dependent. To assure an appropriate time period for bone formation and maturation, a minimum healing period of 6 months is recommended.[6,9] The membrane is removed at abutment surgery (Figs 6-1n to v) if primary wound healing over the membrane has been maintained.

The procedure for using GBR to resolve a dehiscence defect that resulted from insufficient bone volume and ideal implant placement is shown in Figs 6-2a to h.

Dehiscence defects.   *Figs 6-1a to v*

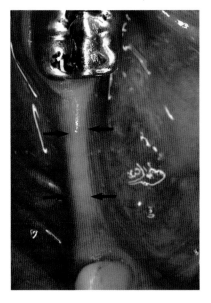 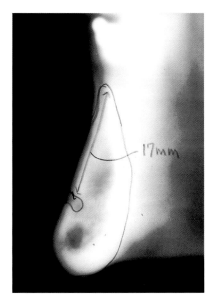

6-1a   **6-1b**

Flap design and procedure

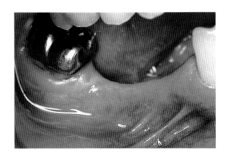 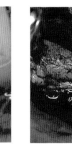

6-1c   **6-1d**   **6-1e**

Fig 6-1a   Partial edentulous space in the right mandible. Clinical examination demonstrates an insufficient crest width *(arrows)* for standard implant placement.

Fig 6-1b   Conventional tomogram reveals the narrow alveolar crest and an adequate vertical bone height of 17 mm above the mandibular canal.

Fig 6-1c   Buccal view of the edentulous space in the right mandible. Healthy soft tissue conditions are present.

Fig 6-1d   Remote flap design using a superficial incision of the mucosa at the buccal aspect 3 to 4 mm apical to the mucogingival junction.

Fig 6-1e   Elevation of the combined split-thickness/full-thickness flap to the lingual aspect. The buccal periosteal flap is not yet elevated (arrows).

Implant and membrane placement

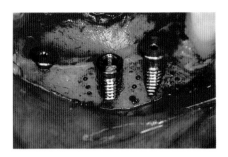

6-1f

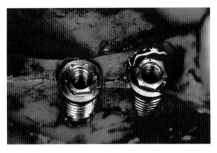

6-1g

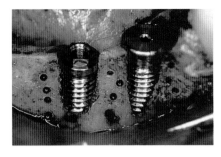

6-1h

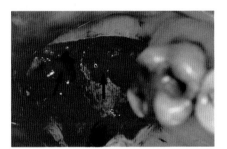

6-1i

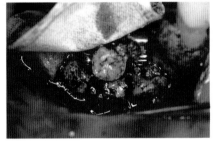

6-1j

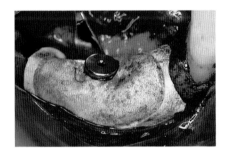

6-1k

Fig 6-1f Placement of three Brånemark implants into the narrow mandibular ridge resulting in extended dehiscence-type defects for the two implants in area 44 and 45. All implants have good primary stability. Note the intact lingual periosteal layer, due to an atraumatic flap elevation, and the buccal bone surface freed from any soft tissue remnants.

Fig 6-1g Occlusal close-up view of two of the implants clearly demonstrates the extended bone defect outside the alveolar housing requiring the use of autogenous bone grafts for space maintenance between the membrane and the implant.

Fig 6-1h Buccal close-up view of two of the implants reveals the extended defects with 8 and 10 threads, respectively, exposed. Note the perforation of the cortical bone plate with a small round bur to open the marrow space, achieving a bleeding bone surface.

Fig 6-1i Donor site in the right tuberosity after harvesting corticocancellous bone grafts with a trephine *(arrows)*.

Fig 6-1j Autogenous corticocancellous bone grafts cover the exposed implant surfaces to stabilize the blood clot and to maintain the space between the membrane and implants.

Fig 6-1k An e-PTFE membrane (GTAM Oval-9) in its final position stabilized by a cover screw. Note the bulk underneath the membrane due to the bone graft and the close adaptation of the membrane in the periphery of the defect.

Wound closure

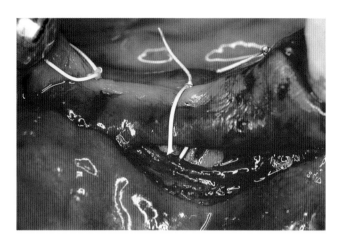

6-1l

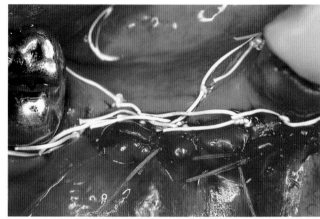

6-1m

Healing period

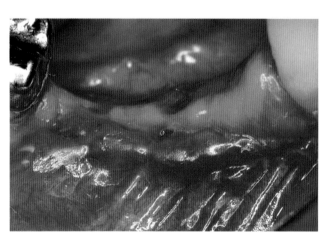

6-1n

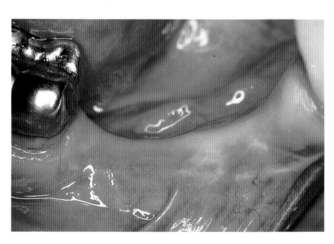

6-1o

Fig 6-1l   Initiation of wound closure with three mattress sutures approximating the lingual flap with the buccal periosteum.

Fig 6-1m   Completion of a tension-free primary soft tissue closure with horizontal mattress and interrupted sutures.

Fig 6-1n   Clinical status 3 weeks after membrane surgery and immediately after suture removal.

Fig 6-1o   Clinical status 6 months after membrane surgery with a complete soft tissue coverage of the membrane site.

Membrane removal

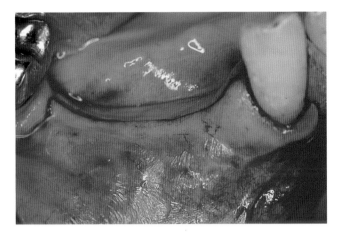

6-1p

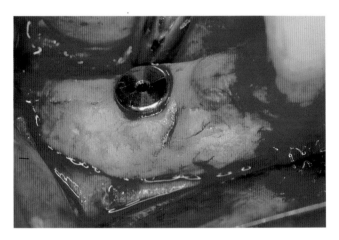

6-1q

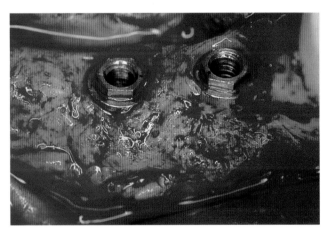

6-1r

Fig 6-1p   Midcrestal incision at the second-stage surgery 6 months following membrane placement.

Fig 6-1q   Intrasurgical status at reopening demonstrates the membrane in proper position with a typical transparent appearance.

Fig 6-1r   Following membrane removal, the previous dehiscence defects are completely regenerated with newly formed bone.

Post-treatment status

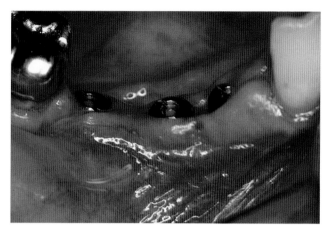

6-1s

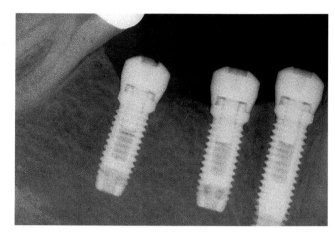

6-1t

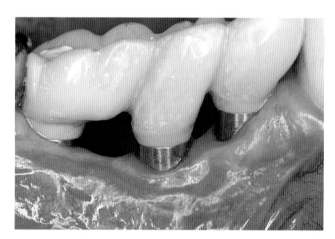

6-1u

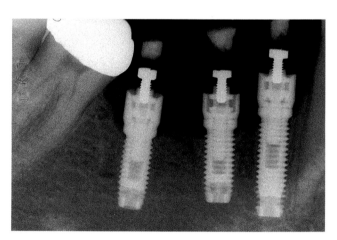

6-1v

Fig 6-1s Clinical status 3 weeks after abutment placement. The soft and hard tissues were allowed to mature with transgingival abutments without functional loading for a total of 2 months.

Fig 6-1t Periapical radiograph following abutment connection demonstrates normal bone structures around the three implants.

Fig 6-1u Clinical status of acrylic resin provisional prosthesis placed on implants 2 months after second-stage surgery.

Fig 6-1v Periapical radiograph showing peri-implant bone structures 6 months after second-stage surgery.

Ideal implant placement resulting in dehiscence defect.
Figs 6-2a to h

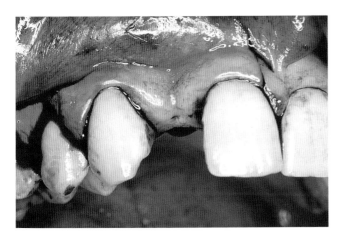

6-2a

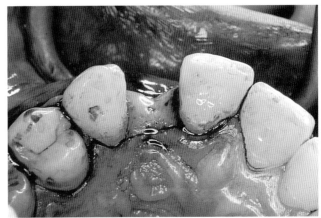

6-2b

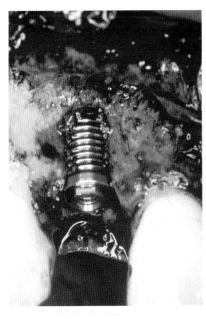

6-2c

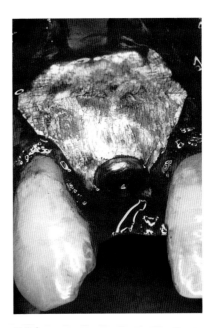

6-2d

Fig 6-2a Sulcular incision and distal line angle releasing incisions in a single-tooth gap in the maxilla.

Fig 6-2b Occlusal view demonstrates the remote flap design with a beveled palatal incision technique.

Fig 6-2c Ideal implant placement resulted in a superficial dehiscence defect with nine exposed implant threads.

Fig 6-2d Placement of an e-PTFE membrane (GTAM Oval-6) stabilized by a cover screw and trimmed to utilize the stiffer inner portion of the membrane and the adjacent root emergences for spacemaking.

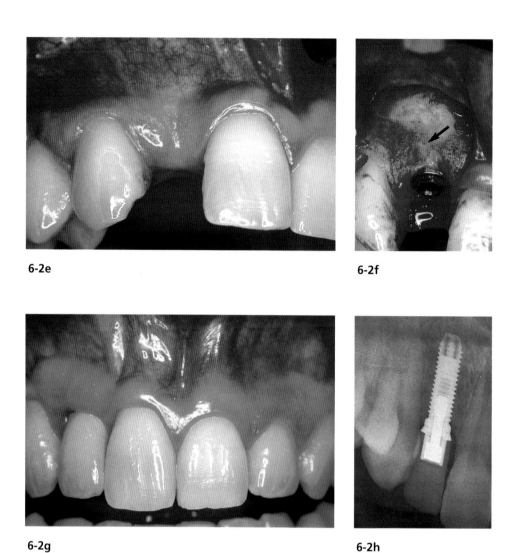

6-2e

6-2f

6-2g

6-2h

Fig 6-2e Clinical status after a complication-free healing period of 6 months.

Fig 6-2f Intrasurgical status following membrane removal. The previous dehiscence defect is regenerated with newly formed bone and a thin superficial soft tissue layer *(arrow)*.

Fig 6-2g Clinical status 12 months after implant placement and restoration with a full ceramic crown on a Cera-One abutment. (Restorative treatment by Dr Hans Kelderman, Harvard University School of Dentistry.)

Fig 6-2h Periapical radiograph 12 months after implant placement demonstrates regular peri-implant bone structures.

Short-term results with a 1- to 3-year follow-up on implants with membrane-regenerated bone demonstrated an increased bone loss during the first year with a stable situation thereafter. It was found that the peri-implant bone loss after 1 year of prosthesis function was 1.7 mm.[6,31] Until more long-term data on the stability of regenerated bone tissue are available and the regeneration process is fully understood, it seems reasonable to suggest that implants be gradually loaded to allow the bone time to become fully loadbearing.[32]

The following protocol is currently being utilized:

1. After second-stage surgery, the peri-implant soft and hard tissues are allowed to mature with transgingival abutments without functional loading.
2. Approximately 2 months after second-stage surgery, implant loading is initiated with the use of a provisional prosthesis made of acrylic resin.
3. Six to 9 months following second-stage surgery, the implants are restored with a fixed prosthesis.

An exception to this protocol is made for implants placed in the edentulous maxilla to retain an overdenture with bar-clip attachments. These implants are connected by a bar soon after second-stage surgery.

Guided Bone Regeneration in Delayed Extraction Sockets

Maxillary and mandibular premolars, canines, and incisors are ideal candidates for extraction and immediate implant placement when severe periodontal breakdown, root fractures, or endodontic failures are evident.[22] There are four prerequisites:

1. After tooth extraction, the socket must present sufficient residual walls.
2. The extraction socket must be free of pathosis.
3. The available soft tissue should allow primary closure.
4. Apical to the apex of the socket, a sufficient volume of healthy jawbone must be available to assure good initial stabilization of the implant.

Most of the surgical procedures described previously for the treatment of implant sites with a dehiscence defect are identical. However, the mucogingival situation around an extraction socket is often unfavorable to achieve primary closure. Due to the decreased quantity and quality of regenerated tissue when the membrane becomes exposed, a modified surgical protocol is followed to ensure predictable soft tissue coverage over the extraction site.[7,9,23]

After all diagnostic procedures are carefully evaluated, the tooth is planned for extraction. An intrasulcular incision is performed and a mucoperiostal flap around the involved tooth is elevated. Subsequently, the tooth is extracted atraumatically, while preserving the surrounding bone walls. The socket is debrided of granulation tissue with curettes and excavators. The flaps are released and soft tissue closure is achieved with horizontal mattress sutures and interrupted sutures.

An assessment of the root orientation and the size of the extraction defect must be made, since this has a direct influence on the angulation of the implant and the predictability of the regenerative procedure. In situations where the extraction socket is inappropriate to place an implant, the original protocol of a 6- to 12-month healing period to allow complete ossification of the extraction socket, or a staged approach utilizing the GBR technique for localized ridge augmentation (see Chapter 7), is recommended.

In situations where the extraction socket is appropriate for implant placement, the patient is evaluated approximately 8 weeks following extraction for complete soft tissue coverage of the extraction site. When complete coverage has occurred, a remote flap design (as previously described) is initiated. Soft tissue that is present in the coronal half of the socket should be removed. The implant should be placed at least 3 to 4 mm beyond the original apex of the socket to ensure stability (Figs 6-3a to d). Bleeding from the bone preparation should allow the formation of a clot in the space between the exposed implant surface and the socket walls. Complete coverage of the bone-implant voids with the membrane is essential to prevent any ingrowth of gingival connective tissue (Fig 6-3e). The flap management and suturing technique should allow for primary flap closure even if there is a risk of creating scar bands. If scar bands occur, they can be easily corrected at membrane removal by applying mucogingival surgery techniques to the peri-implant tissue. Postsurgical controls will detect any wound healing problems, and membrane exposure will automatically mean its early removal. Further procedures are the same as those described for dehisced implant sites (Figs 6-3f to j).

Delayed extraction sockets.   *Figs 6-3a to j*

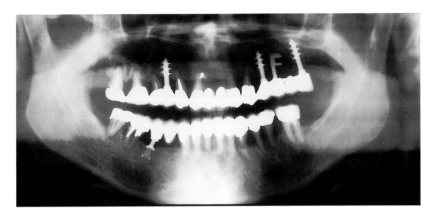

6-3a

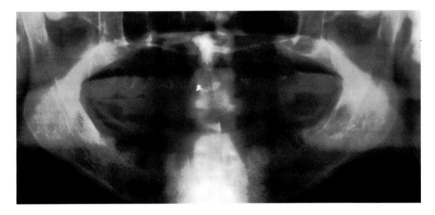

6-3b

Fig 6-3a Panoramic radiograph demonstrates severe adult periodontitis as well as several failing implants in the maxilla and the mandible requiring implant and tooth removal.

Fig 6-3b Panoramic radiograph after removal of all remaining teeth and implants.

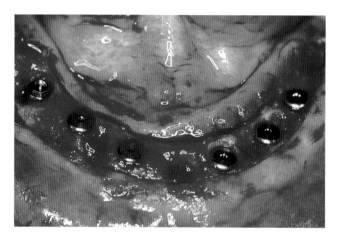

6-3c

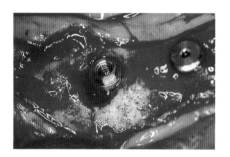

6-3d

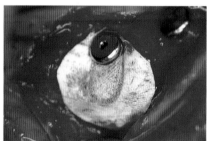

6-3e

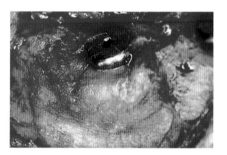

6-3f

Fig 6-3c   Two months after extraction and complete soft tissue healing, six Brånemark implants are placed in the edentulous mandible.

Fig 6-3d   Close-up view of the implant placed in a delayed extraction socket (area 44). The implant site demonstrates a peri-implant bone defect that is space-maintaining.

Fig 6-3e   Placement of an e-PTFE membrane covering the peri-implant bone defect. The membrane is stabilized by the cover screw.

Fig 6-3f   Clinical status 6 months after a complication-free soft tissue healing and reopening of the site. The membrane is still in place and demonstrates a close adaptation to the underlying newly regenerated tissues.

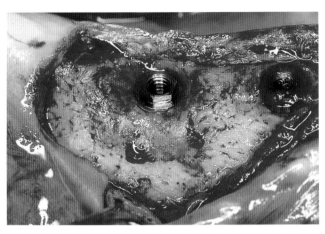

6-3g

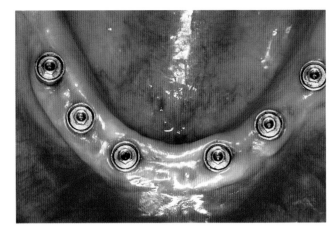

6-3h

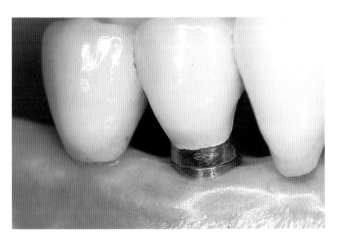

6-3i

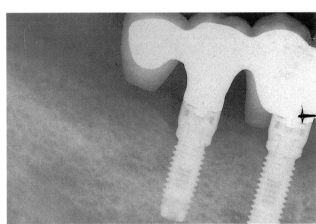

6-3j

Fig 6-3g Buccal view of the implant site in area 44 after membrane removal. The bone defect is completely filled with newly formed bone.

Fig 6-3h Clinical status after abutment connection and excellent soft tissue healing. Note the good anteroposterior distribution of the six implants.

Fig 6-3i Clinical status 12 months after implant placement and restoration with a fixed partial denture. (Restorative treatment by Dr Dirk Braakman, Utrecht, The Netherlands.)

Fig 6-3j Periapical radiograph 12 months after implant placement demonstrates regular peri-implant bone structures.

Simultaneous Use of Guided Bone Regeneration With ITI Implants

The surgical procedure for the simultaneous application of e-PTFE (GTAM) membranes and ITI implants (Institut Straumann AG, Waldenburg, Switzerland) does not differ from the procedure with Brånemark implants described earlier in this chapter. However, the surgical procedure differs from the standard implant placement of ITI implants, since they were originally designed to be nonsubmerged implants.[12,33] ITI implants have been characterized by a nonsubmerged, transgingival healing since 1974, when the first prototypes were developed and clinical testing began in patients. Therefore, ITI implants are utilized in standard situations with a one-stage surgical procedure, avoiding a second-stage surgery.[17] In special situations, such as in combination with iliac bone grafts in extremely atrophied edentulous jaws[34] or with barrier membranes,[3,8,9] ITI implants are submerged underneath the soft tissue to protect the membrane against the bacteria of the oral cavity. Special consideration has to be given to the placement of ITI implants in these situations.

The initial incision technique and flap design are the same as described previously; a lateral incision technique is used on the palatal aspect in the maxilla (Figs 6-4a and b) or on the buccal aspect for mandibular sites. Emphasis is given to a large base of the combined split-thickness/full-thickness flap to provide a sufficient vascular supply for the flap by means of divergent vertical relieving incisions. Following intrasurgical examination of the local bone anatomy, the ultimate decision between a simultaneous or staged approach is made. If a simultaneous approach is chosen, the implant recipient site and the appropriate ITI implant type are selected. The ITI system consists of three different implant types: the solid-screw (standard and diameter-reduced versions), the hollow-screw, and the hollow-cylinder (straight and with a 15-degree angulation). In dehiscence-type defects in the crest area, all three implant types can theoretically be used, as long as sufficient primary stability can be achieved. However, in combination with barrier membranes, the hollow-cylinder implant is only used in its angled version if a correction of the implant axis is necessary; this is often the case for single-tooth replacements in the anterior maxilla. Otherwise, threaded implants are usually preferred. The selection for one of the two threaded implants available is made depending on the vertical bone height present. If a long implant (from 10 to 16 mm) can be inserted, the solid-screw is the implant of choice. If a short implant (6 to 8 mm) must be used because of a reduced vertical bone height, preference is given to a hollow-screw implant with its increased anchoring surface in the "apical" portion. In fenestration-type defects, use of a solid-screw implant is recommended, because the open basket of hollow-cylinder or hollow-screw implants should not be exposed to the defect area.

The implant recipient site is prepared with standard ITI instruments for harvesting of autogenous bone grafts from the recipient site. One such procedure uses the standard trephine to create a bone core inside the recipient site (Fig 6-4c). This bone core can be fractured and removed from the site (Fig 6-4d), then cut with a rongeur (Fig 6-4e) into small bone chips, which are stored in sterile saline before graft application (Fig 6-4f). The spiral drills of the ITI system offer another method for harvesting bone grafts (Figs 6-4g and h). The sink depth is calculated as the length of the selected implant (length of the plasma-sprayed implant coating) plus 2 mm. This simple calculation allows placement of the implant deep enough into the bone to close the mucosa primarily and leaves the implant shoulder approximately 1 mm above the crest level. As a consequence, the crestal portion of the bone cavity has to be prepared with a special countersink drill (Fig 6-4i). The implant is inserted to the predetermined sink depth and the extent of the exposed implant surface is examined (Fig 6-4j). For peri-implant bone defects outside the alveolar housing, autogenous bone grafts are now routinely used as a membrane-supporting device for space maintenance as well as an osteoconductive scaffold to accelerate bone regeneration. If necessary, additional bone grafts are harvested in the periapical area of the implant with a chisel (Fig 6-4k). Following perforation of the surrounding cortical bone plate to open the marrow space and to achieve a bleeding bone surface, the bone grafts are placed in the site to cover the exposed implant surface (Fig 6-4l).

Subsequently, the membrane is trimmed with scissors as outlined above (Fig 6-4m). Emphasis is given to the stabilization of the membrane. The membrane is primarily stabilized with fixation screws of the Memfix System (Institut Straumann AG). The membrane is punched in a proper position, applied to the site with the curved end of the membrane placement instrument (Hu-Friedy, Chicago; Fig 6-4n), and stabilized with the spike end of the same instrument (Fig 6-4o). Subsequently, the bone is prepared with the special Memfix drill (Fig 6-4p) to allow insertion of the self-tapping fixation screw with the special screwdriver (Fig 6-4q). In sites with a thick soft tissue cover, the membrane is also stabilized on top of the implant shoulder with a large healing cap (Figs 6-4r to t). The large healing cap should not be used in sites with a thin soft tissue cover. In these sites, the small healing cap is preferred to protect the inner portion of the implant against soft tissue ingrowth during healing. A hole with a diameter of 4.2 mm is punched into the membrane in proper position (Fig 6-4u). Subsequently, the membrane with its punched hole is placed around the neck of the implant shoulder. This simple procedure also stabilizes the membrane sufficiently (Figs 6-4v and w). Wound closure is achieved with the same suturing technique as described above (Figs 6-4t and x).

The technique described is demonstrated in three patients, two of them with implants in the maxilla (Figs 6-5a to l and Figs 6-6a to l) and one with an implant in the mandible (Figs 6-7a to l).

Technique for simultancous use of GBR with ITI implants.
Figs 6-4a to x

Lateral incision technique

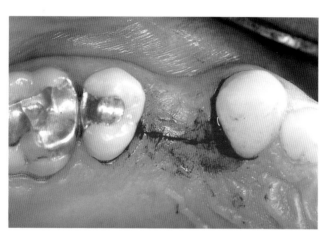

6-4a

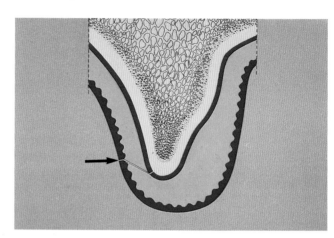

6-4b

Fig 6-4a   Lateral incision technique at the palatal aspect in a single tooth gap in area 14.

Fig 6-4b   Schematic drawing of the lateral incision technique in the maxilla using a split-thickness incision of the mucosa *(arrow)* and a supra-periosteal flap preparation toward the crest.

Fig 6-4c   Preparation of the implant recipient site with an ITI trephine creating a bone core *(arrow)* to be used as an autogenous bone graft. Fine bone chips can also be harvested from the bone surface with a surgical curette.

Fig 6-4d   Bone core harvested from a recipient site prepared with a trephine.

Fig 6-4e   Rongeur is used to cut the bone core into smaller bone chips.

Fig 6-4f   Prior to graft application, the bone chips are stored in sterile saline.

Fig 6-4g   Pilot drills of the ITI system provide an alternative method for harvesting autogenous bone grafts from an implant recipient site. Note the bone chips inside the thread of the pilot drill *(arrow)*.

Fig 6-4h   Fine bone chips are removed from the spiral drill with a periodontal probe and stored in sterile saline.

Bone harvesting—method 1

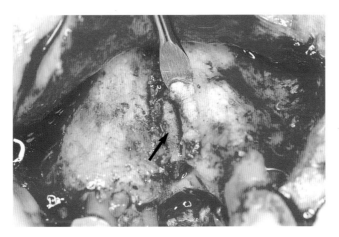

6-4c

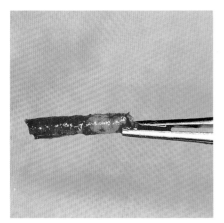

6-4d

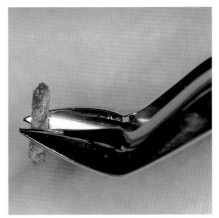

6-4e

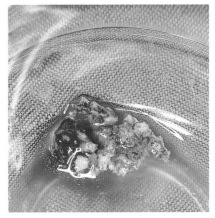

6-4f

Bone harvesting—method 2

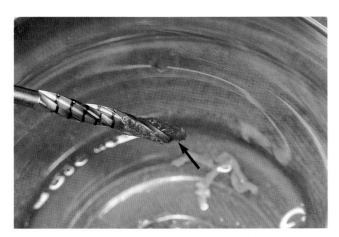

6-4g

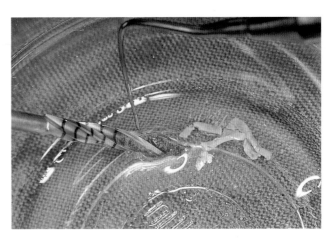

6-4h

Implant and graft placement

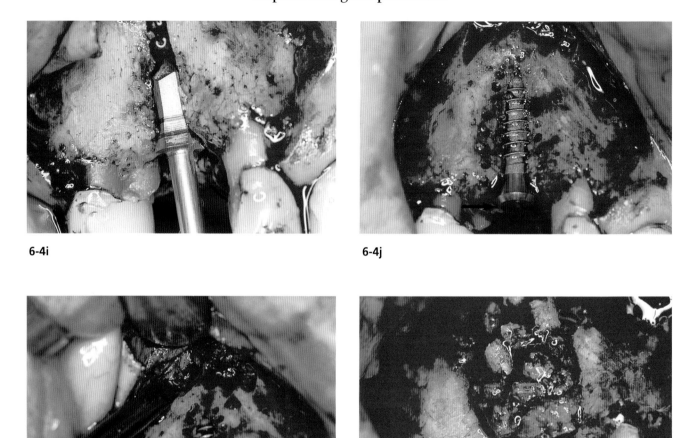

6-4i

6-4j

6-4k

6-4l

Fig 6-4i Preparation of the crestal portion of the recipient site with an ITI countersink drill. This drill has two lines to facilitate the correct determination of the sink depth.

Fig 6-4j Status following placement of a solid-screw implant in area 13. The implant is inserted deeper into the bone than in a standard situation, allowing primary wound closure. The implant shoulder *(arrow)* is located approximately 1 mm above the alveolar crest. Note the extended dehiscence-type defect with a completely exposed implant surface.

Fig 6-4k Harvesting of additional bone grafts in the "periapical" area with a round chisel.

Fig 6-4l Application of the bone grafts to cover the exposed implant surface. The autogenous bone grafts serve as a space-maintaining device and osteoconductive scaffold.

Membrane placement and stabilization

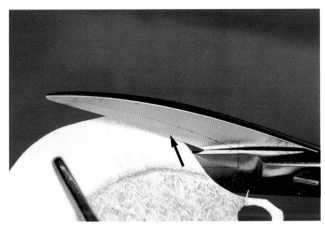

6-4m

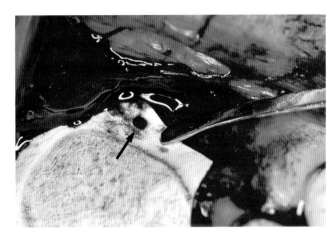

6-4n

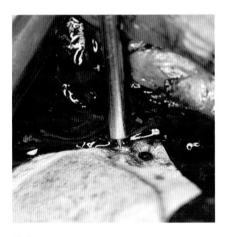

6-4o

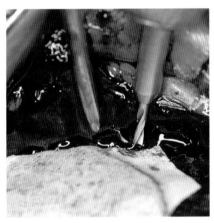

6-4p

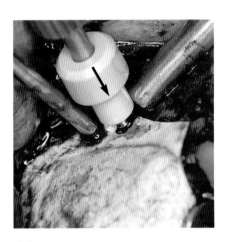

6-4q

Fig 6-4m Membrane is trimmed with scissors with carbide inserts *(arrows)*.

Fig 6-4n Punched membrane *(arrow)* is applied to the site with the curved end of the membrane placement instrument (Hu-Friedy, Chicago, IL) to achieve a close adaptation of the membrane to the bone surface.

Fig 6-4o Membrane is secured in place with the spike end of the membrane placement instrument.

Fig 6-4p Memfix drill is used to prepare a hole through the punched perforation into the bone for the fixation screw.

Fig 6-4q Insertion of the self-tapping fixation screw with the screwdriver *(arrow)* for membrane stabilization and adaptation to the bone.

Large healing cap—thick soft tissue cover

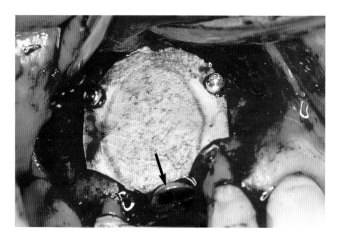

6-4r

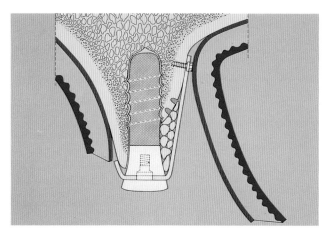

6-4s

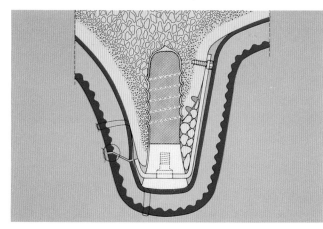

6-4t

Fig 6-4r Stabilization of the membrane with two fixation screws and with a large healing cap *(arrow)*.

Fig 6-4s Schematic drawing of membrane application stabilized on top of the implant with a large healing cap and fixation screws in the "apical" area. Note the bone chips supporting the membrane.

Fig 6-4t Schematic drawing of primary wound closure with mattress and interrupted sutures.

Small healing cap—thin soft tissue cover

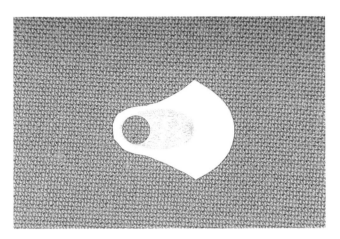

6-4u

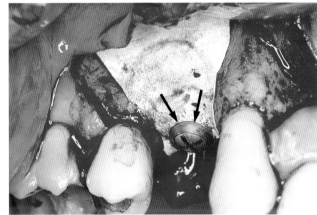

6-4v

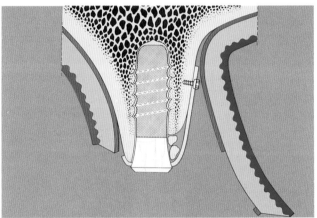

6-4w

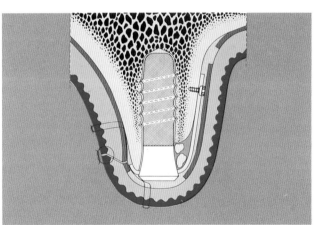

6-4x

Fig 6-4u Perforation of the trimmed membrane with the 4.2-mm punch to be adapted around the neck of the implant.

Fig 6-4v Application of the membrane around the neck of the implant *(arrows)* to stabilize the membrane.

Fig 6-4w Schematic drawing of membrane application around the neck of the implant. The membrane is secured in place by the implant and a fixation screw.

Fig 6-4x Schematic drawing of primary wound closure with mattress and interrupted sutures.

Patient 1

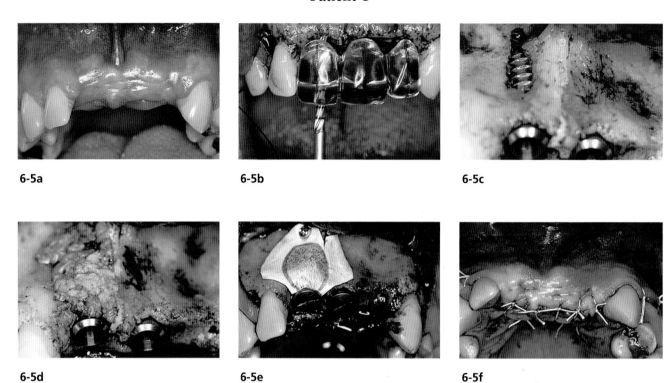

6-5a

6-5b

6-5c

6-5d

6-5e

6-5f

Fig 6-5a Clinical status following traumatic loss of three teeth in the anterior maxilla.

Fig 6-5b Preparation of the recipient site for two implants using a surgical stent for proper positioning and correct implant axis.

Fig 6-5c The correct implant placement from a prosthetic point of view results in a buccal fenestration-type defect with six threads exposed.

Fig 6-5d Application of autogenous bone grafts harvested from the two implant recipient sites.

Fig 6-5e Application of e-PTFE membrane to cover the defect and the bone grafts. The membrane is secured by a large healing cap and one fixation screw in the area of the nasal spine.

Fig 6-5f Primary wound closure by two horizontal mattress sutures and several interrupted sutures.

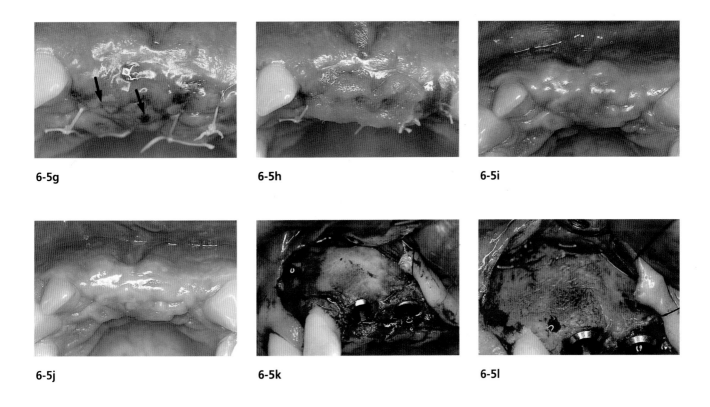

6-5g   **6-5h**   **6-5i**

6-5j   **6-5k**   **6-5l**

Fig 6-5g   Clinical status 1 week after membrane surgery. Note the superficial necrosis of the epithelium *(arrows)*.

Fig 6-5h   Local application of Solcoseryl dental adhesive paste (Soeco Basel AG, Birsfelden, Switzerland) to foster soft tissue healing by granulation.

Fig 6-5i   Clinical status 3 weeks after membrane surgery. The soft tissues are superficially healed.

Fig 6-5j   Clinical status at the end of the complication-free healing period of 6 months.

Fig 6-5k   Reopening status 6 months after membrane surgery. The membrane is still in place.

Fig 6-5l   Intrasurgical status following membrane removal demonstrates complete regeneration of the defect with newly formed bone.

Patient 2

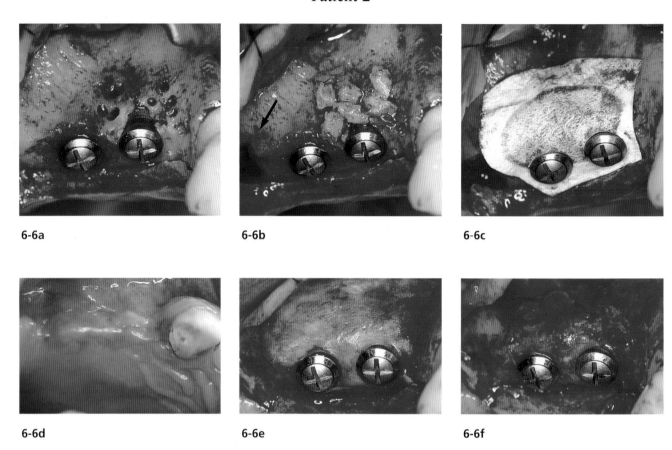

6-6a

6-6b

6-6c

6-6d

6-6e

6-6f

Fig 6-6a   Placement of two ITI implants in the posterior edentulous area of the right maxilla. The implants are placed deeper into the bone, locating the implant shoulder slightly above the crest surface. The implant in area 14 demonstrated a buccal dehiscence defect.

Fig 6-6b   Application of autogenous bone grafts to cover the defect and the exposed implant surface. The grafts were harvested more distally *(arrow)* with a chisel.

Fig 6-6c   Placement of e-PTFE membrane with two punched perforations. The membrane is stabilized by the neck of the two implants and closely adapted to the surrounding bone surface.

Fig 6-6d   Clinical status after a complication-free healing period of 6 months without soft tissue dehiscence and membrane exposure.

Fig 6-6e   Status at second-stage surgery with the membrane still in a proper position.

Fig 6-6f   Status following membrane removal demonstrates complete osseous healing of the previously existing bone defect.

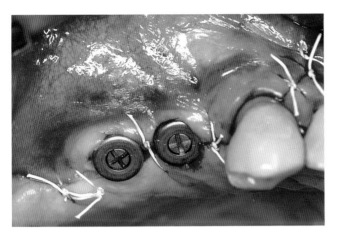

6-6g

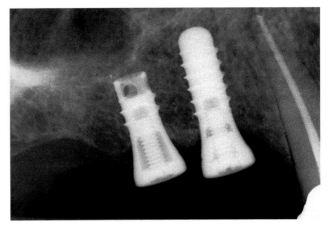

6-6h

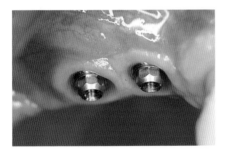

6-6i

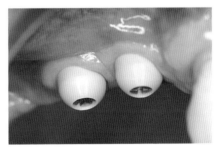

6-6j

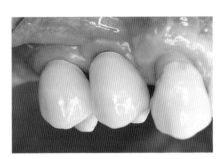

6-6k

Fig 6-6g   Precise wound closure after application of 2-mm transgingival healing caps and close adaptation of the wound margins to these caps.

Fig 6-6h   Periapical radiograph after second-stage surgery demonstrates the 6-mm hollow-screw and the 10-mm solid-screw implants with regular peri-implant bone structures.

Fig 6-6i   Clinical status after soft tissue healing of 6 weeks and insertion of two Octa-abutments for prosthetic restoration.

Fig 6-6j   Application of two plastic healing caps to maintain the soft tissue contour.

Fig 6-6k   Clinical status 12 months after implant placement. The two implants are restored with two single crowns. (Prosthetic restorations by Dr M. Lamparter, Aarwangen, Switzerland.)

Fig 6-6l   Periapical radiograph 12 months after implant placement demonstrates normal bone structures around the 6-mm hollow-screw implant and the 10-mm solid-screw implant.

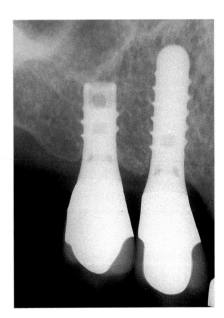

6-6l

Patient 3

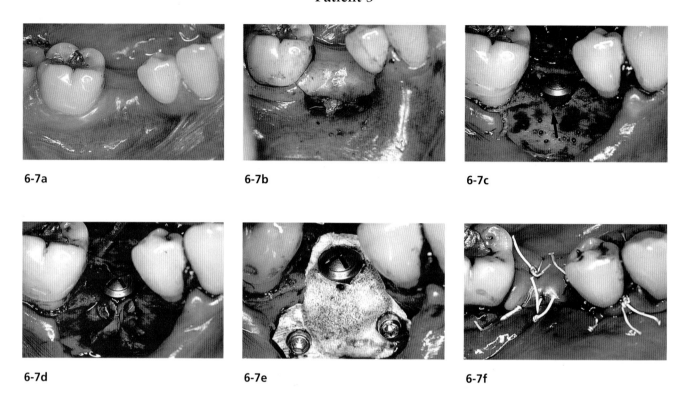

6-7a   6-7b   6-7c

6-7d   6-7e   6-7f

Fig 6-7a   Single-tooth gap in the right mandible.

Fig 6-7b   Buccal split-thickness incision of the mucosa with a subsequent supraperiosteal preparation to the crest and incision of the periosteum at the level of the mucogingival junction.

Fig 6-7c   Status after placement of an 8-mm ITI implant to a sink depth of approximately 10 mm. Note the buccal dehiscence defect of approximately 3 mm and the thin buccal bone plate *(arrow)*.

Fig 6-7d   Application of autogenous bone grafts harvested in the right retromolar area.

Fig 6-7e   Placement of e-PTFE membrane (GTAM Oval-6) stabilized by two fixation screws in a more apical area. The punched membrane is further stabilized around the neck of the implant.

Fig 6-7f   Primary wound closure is obtained by two vertical mattress sutures and several interrupted sutures.

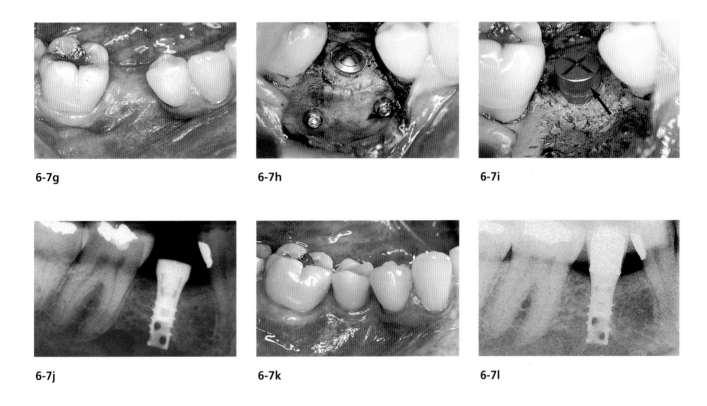

6-7g 6-7h 6-7i

6-7j 6-7k 6-7l

Fig 6-7g Clinical status 6 months after complication-free soft tissue healing.

Fig 6-7h Intrasurgical status at second-stage surgery with the membrane still in a proper position.

Fig 6-7i Status following membrane removal. The previously existing bone defect is filled with newly formed bone, establishing a new buccal bone wall of sufficient thickness. As planned, the implant shoulder *(arrow)* is located 1 mm above the bone crest.

Fig 6-7j Periapical radiograph after second-stage surgery demonstrates regular bone structures around the 8-mm hollow-screw implant.

Fig 6-7k Clinical status following restoration of the implant with a metal ceramic single crown. (Prosthetic treatment by Dr Sandro Leoncini, University of Berne; laboratory work by Mr B. Heckendorn, Labor Busch, Bern, Switzerland.)

Fig 6-7l Periapical radiograph 15 months after implant placement reveals normal peri-implant bone structures and the precision between the implant and the restoration.

Membrane Exposure

If a soft tissue dehiscence occurs during the healing period and the membrane becomes exposed to the intraoral environment, a maintenance problem develops. As a consequence, the membrane will be contaminated by microorganisms from the oral cavity.[35,36] To decrease the risk of an acute infection with purulent flow in the exposed membrane site, the patient is placed on a strict antimicrobial regimen including local rinsing with chlorhexidine. Furthermore, the patient is seen by the clinician on a weekly basis to examine the membrane site. During these recall visits, the area of the exposed membrane is carefully debrided. If no signs of an exudate become evident, the membrane is left in place up to 8 weeks following placement and then removed. If the site develops an exudate or purulent drainage, immediate removal of the membrane is recommended. At this surgery, a flap is raised and the infected membrane must be totally removed. Then the site is thoroughly irrigated with chlorhexidine (0.12%), and the regenerated tissue found underneath the barrier (usually reddish granulation tissue) is left undisturbed, since it might still have some osteogenic potential. Care is taken to de-epithelialize the margins of the flap with sharp dissection and to close the flap over the newly regenerated tissue without tension. Thereafter, a minimum healing period of 6 months from membrane placement is recommended. Depending on the defect size and morphology at the time of implant placement, the occurrence of an exposed membrane will influence the amount of bone formation.[2,6] Premature membrane removal can result in excessive soft tissue shrinkage and undesirable clinical results.

Summary

Based on more than 5 years of clinical experience, the simultaneous application of barrier membranes for the treatment of peri-implant bone defects has shown predictable and significant formation of new bone. The clinical results of this surgically sensitive technique are dependent on flap design and flap management during surgery, bone bed preparation, creation and maintenance of a space between the implant and the inner surface of the membrane, stabilization of the membrane, as well as an undisturbed submerged healing of the membrane for 4 to 6 months depending on the defect size.

Acknowledgment

The authors thank Mrs Oedipe for drawing the schematic diagrams.

References

1. Newman M, Flemmig T. Periodontal considerations of implants and implant-associated microbiota. J Dent Educ 1988;52:737.

2. Lazzara R. Immediate implant placement into extraction sites. Surgical and restorative advantages. Int J Periodont Rest Dent 1989;9:33.

3. Nyman S, Lang NP, Buser D, Brägger U. Bone regeneration adjacent to titanium dental implants using guided tissue regeneration: A report of two cases. Int J Oral Maxillofac Implants 1990;5:9.

4. Becker W, Becker BE. Guided tissue regeneration for implants placed into extraction sockets and for implant dehiscences: Surgical techniques and case reports. Int J Periodont Rest Dent 1990;10:377.

5. Dahlin C, Andersson L, Linde A. Bone augmentation at fenestrated implants by an osteopromotive membrane technique. A controlled clinical study. Clin Oral Impl Res 1991;2:159.

6. Jovanovic SA, Spiekermann H, Richter EJ. Bone regeneration on titanium dental implants with dehisced defect sites. A clinical study. Int J Oral Maxillofac Implants 1992;7:233.

7. Jovanovic SA, Spiekermann H, Richter EJ, Koseoglu M. Guided tissue regeneration around titanium dental implants. In: Laney WR, Tolman DE (eds). Tissue Integration in Oral, Orthopedic, and Maxillofacial Reconstruction. Chicago: Quintessence, 1992:208–215.

8. Weingart D, Biggel A. Lokale periimplantäre Augmentation des anterioren Unterkiefer-Alveolarfortsatzes nach dem Prinzip der gesteuerten Geweberegeneration (GTR). Quintessenz 1992;43:403.

9. Buser D, Hirt HP, Dula K, Berthold H. Membrantechnik-Orale Implantologie: Gleichzeitige Anwendung von Membranen bei Implantaten mit periimplantären Knochendefekten. Schweiz Monatsschr Zahnmed 1992;102:1491.

10. Kenney EB, Jovanovic SA. Osteopromotion as an adjunct to osseointegration. Int J Prosthodont 1993;6:131.

11. Schenk RK, Willenegger H. Zur Histologie der primären Knochenheilung. Modifikationen und Grenzen der Spaltheilung in Abhängigkeit von der Defektgrösse. Unfallheilkunde 1977;80:155.

12. Buser D, Schroeder A, Sutter F, Lang NP. The new concept of ITI hollow-cylinder and hollow-screw implants: Part 2. Clinical aspects, indications, and early clinical results. Int J Oral Maxillofac Implants 1988;3:173.

13. Schwarz MS, Rothman SLG, Rhodes ML, Chafetz N. Computed tomography: Part 1: Preoperative assessment of the mandible for endosseous implant surgery. Int J Oral Maxillofac Implants 1987;2:137.

14. Kassebaum DK, Nummikoski PV, Triplett RG, Langlais RP. Cross-sectional radiography for implant site assessment. Oral Surg Oral Med Oral Pathol 1990;70:674.

15. Buser D, Dula K, Belser U, Hirt HP, Berthold H. Localized ridge augmentation using guided bone regeneration. I. Surgical procedure in the maxilla. Int J Periodont Rest Dent 1993;13:29.

16. Carlsson GE, Persson G. Morphologic changes of the mandible after extraction and wearing of dentures. A longitudinal, clinical and x-ray cephalometric study covering 5 years. Odontol Rev 1967;18:27.

17. Mecall RA, Rosenfeld AI. The influence of residual ridge resorption patterns on implant fixture placement and tooth position. Int J Periodont Rest Dent 1991;11:19.

18. Buser D, Brägger U, Lang NP, Nyman S. Regeneration and enlargement of jaw bone using guided tissue regeneration. Clin Oral Impl Res 1990;1:22.

19. Shanaman RH. The use of guided tissue regeneration to facilitate ideal prosthetic placement of implants. Int J Periodont Rest Dent 1992;12:257.

20. Gotfredsen K, Warrer K, Hjørting-Hansen E, Karring T. Effect of membranes and hydroxyapatite on healing in bone defects around titanium implants. An experimental study in the monkey. Clin Oral Impl Res 1991;2:172.

21. Caudill RF, Meffert RM. Histologic analysis of the osseointegration of endosseous implants in simulated extraction sockets with and without e-PTFE barriers. Part 1: Preliminary findings. Int J Periodont Rest Dent 1991;11:207.

22. Wachtel HC, Langford A, Bernimoulin JP, Reichart P. Guided bone regeneration next to osseointegrated implants in humans. Int J Oral Maxillofac Implants 1991;2:127.

23. Jovanovic SA, Giovanoli JL. New bone formation by the principle of guided tissue regeneration for peri-implant osseous lesions. J Parodontologie 1992;11:29.

24. Habal MB, Reddi AH. Bone Grafts and Bone Substitutes. Philadelphia: Saunders, 1992.

25. Beresford JN. Osteogenic stem cells and the stromal system of bone and marrow. Clin Orthop 1989;240:270.

26. Wlodarski KH. Properties and origin of osteoblasts. Clin Orthop 1990;252:276.

27. Mizuno K, Mineo K, Tachibana T, et al. The osteogenic potential of fracture hematoma. Subperiosteal and intramuscular transplantation of the haematoma. J Bone Joint Surg 1990;72:822.

28. Vargerik K, Ousterhout DK. Clinical and experimental bone formation. Adv Plast Reconstr Surg 1987;4:95.

29. Skoog T. The use of periosteum and Surgicel for bone restoration in congenital clefts of the maxilla. Scand J Plast Reconstr Surg 1967;1:113.

30. Brunksi JB, Moccia AF, Pollack SR, et al. The influence of functional use of endosseous dental implants on the tissue-implant interface. J Dent Res 1979;58:1953.

31. Dahlin C, Lekholm U, Linde A. Membrane induced bone augmentation at titanium implants. Int J Periodont Rest Dent 1991;11:273.

32. Roberts WE, Smith RK, Zilberman Y, et al. Remodeling of devitalized bone threatens periosteal integrity of endosseous titanium implants with threaded or smooth surfaces: Indications for provisional loading and axillary directed occlusion. J Indiana Dent Assoc 1989;68:95.

33. Sutter F, Schroeder A, Buser D. The new concept of ITI hollow-cylinder and hollow-screw implants: Part 1. Engineering and design. Int J Oral Maxillofac Implants 1988;3:161.

34. Weingart D, Strub JR, Schilli W. Mandibular ridge augmentation with autogenous bone grafts and immediate implants. A 3-year longitudinal study [abstract 105]. In: Lill W, Spiekermann H, Watzek G (eds). 5th International Congress on Preprosthetic Surgery. Berlin: Quintessence, 1993:119.

35. Selvig KA, Nilveus R, Fitzmorris L, et al. Scanning electron microscopic observations of cell populations and bacterial contamination of membranes used for guided tissue regeneration. J Periodontol 1990;61:515.

36. Tempro PJ, Nalbandian J. Colonization of retrieved polytetrafluoroethylene membranes: Morphological and microbiological observations. J Periodontol 1993;64:162.

CHAPTER SEVEN

Localized Ridge Augmentation Using Guided Bone Regeneration

Daniel Buser
Karl Dula
Hans-Peter Hirt
Hermann Berthold

Localized ridge augmentation prior to the placement of dental implants is one of the clinical indications of guided bone regeneration (GBR) in implant dentistry. This surgical technique using a staged approach (Fig 7-1) is an alternative for the simultaneous approach used in extraction socket defects, dehiscence defects, or fenestration defects (see Chapters 5 and 6). The surgical approach is determined by the presurgical evaluation and, ultimately, by the intrasurgical status, when the ridge anatomy is accessible for a direct examination following flap elevation.

Criteria for Determining the GBR Surgical Approach

1. Primary stability of the implant to be inserted

2. Implant position from a prosthetic point of view

3. Size and type of bone defect

If a potential recipient site does not allow *(1)* the placement of an implant with primary stability or *(2)* the placement of the implant in an appropriate position from a prosthetic point of view, or *(3)* if the bone defect is large and extended, the staged approach for localized ridge augmentation is preferable and offers a more predictable outcome and less risk for the patient.

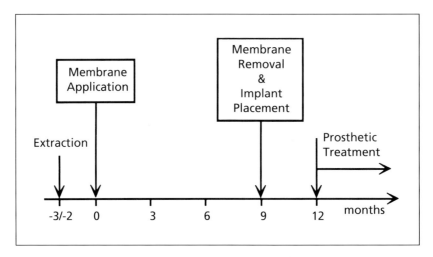

Fig 7-1 Localized ridge augmentation using the GBR technique with a staged approach.

Clinical testing of the GBR technique for localized ridge augmentation using prototype expanded polytetrafluoroethylene (e-PTFE) membranes was initiated at the Department of Oral Surgery, University of Berne, by Professor Sture Nyman in 1988. The results of the first 12 patients treated with the GBR technique for localized ridge augmentation were published in 1990.[1] Based on the clinical experience of these patients, the surgical technique was incrementally modified in 1990/1991 to improve the predictability of the procedure.[2,3] In addition, the successor of the first prototype e-PTFE membranes for implant indications became commercially available in different sizes (Gore-Tex Augmentation Material, GTAM membrane, W.L. Gore, Flagstaff, AZ). This chapter presents the learning experience with localized ridge augmentation during 3 years of development. In particular, problems, complications, and modifications of the surgical technique made during the development period are discussed. The current surgical procedures for indications in the mandible and the maxilla are also detailed.

Development Period From 1988 to 1991

Between November 1988 and July 1989, 12 patients were surgically treated with the GBR technique for localized ridge augmentation (group 1). Some problems during surgery and some complications during the healing period were encountered. The most frequent complications were soft tissue dehiscences. Five patients (41%) demonstrated soft tissue dehiscence and membrane exposure. Three of those patients developed an acute infection with purulent exudate in the surgical site. At the end of the healing period, these three patients demonstrated insufficient bone regeneration for the placement of dental implant(s) in a second surgical procedure. The main reason for this type of complication was an inappropriate incision technique, ie, midcrestal incisions (Figs 7-2a and b) or relieving incisions located directly over or too close to the membrane margin (Figs 7-3a and b). One patient with a midcrestal incision did not develop a soft tissue dehiscence, and this patient demonstrated an excellent ridge augmentation result (Figs 7-4a to j). Based on these observations, the incision technique was changed. Midcrestal incisions were avoided, using instead a lateral incision technique with a combined split-thickness/full-thickness flap design. In addition, vertical relieving incisions were always designed to be 2 to 3 mm from the border of the membrane. This flap design allowed predictable primary soft tissue healing, as well as submerged healing of the membrane without contamination by bacteria from the oral cavity.

One further complication with an acute infection was caused by inappropriate membrane placement; the membrane extended into the sulcus of an adjacent tooth (Figs 7-5a to d). Extension of membranes into sulci of adjacent teeth was subsequently avoided, which left a zone of alveolar bone approximately 1 to 2 mm wide uncovered by the membrane for direct flap attachment.

In the first patients, there also was difficulty stabilizing the membranes and adapting them closely to the surrounding bone surface. This is important to obtain a sealing effect and prevent the ingrowth of competing soft tissue cells from the mucosa. Mini-screws used in maxillofacial surgery for the stabilization of bone fractures were employed for membrane fixation and adaptation, and their use, along with the modified incision technique, resulted in more predictable results. Based on this positive clinical experience, a kit of specially designed mini-screws for membrane fixation and support was developed (Memfix System, Institut Straumann AG, Waldenburg, Switzerland). The kit contains different mini-screws made of stainless steel with an electropolished surface that allows easy removal after a healing period of 9 months. Special instruments were also designed to facilitate the placement of barrier membranes (Figs 7-6a to d).

A further problem was the collapse of the membrane, caused by soft tissue pressure during healing. In the first group of 12 patients, this complication was observed in only one patient with two missing teeth in the maxilla. A few weeks after membrane application, it became obvious from clinical palpation that the membrane had collapsed under the soft tissue cover (Figs 7-7a and b), thus losing the created space. As a consequence, bone regeneration was not sufficient for the placement of implants. Partial membrane collapse was also seen in patients treated within the second group of patients in September 1990. In all of these patients, a collagen sponge (Collagen Fleece, Pentapharm AG,

Basel, Switzerland) was placed under the membranes to stabilize the blood clot in the bone defects (Figs 7-8a and b). After 9 months of healing, partial collapse of the membrane was noted at the buccal aspect of the crest (Figs 7-8c and d). With this collapse, 1 to 2 mm of possible bone gain in crest width was lost. To prevent membrane collapse, supporting screws of the Memfix system were employed as tent poles for the membranes; they were mainly used in extended edentulous spaces (Figs 7-9a to f). The supporting screws were also combined with the collagen sponge as filling material to stabilize the blood clot in the secluded space. Nine months following a complication-free healing (Figs 7-9g and h), reopening still demonstrated a partial membrane collapse lateral to the supporting screw in area 22/23 (Fig 7-9i). The enlargement of the crest width up to 7 mm (Fig 7-9j) allowed the placement of two ITI implants in area 22/23. However, the partial membrane collapse necessitated placement of the implants more toward the palate (Fig 7-9k), resulting in an implant-supported restoration with a ridge lap design (Figs 7-9l to p).

Based on the observation that Collagen Fleece is an excellent blood clot stabilizer but does not have the capacity to support the membrane as a space-maintaining device, the technique was modified once more. It was decided that autogenous bone grafts would be used as a bone filling material and a membrane-supporting device. A young patient with a single-tooth gap in the maxilla was treated in June 1991 with a combination of the GBR technique and autogenous bone grafts (Figs 7-10a and b). The bone graft was harvested from the third molar area in the right mandible and applied to the site to support the membrane (Figs 7-10c to f). After a complication-free healing period of 9 months (Figs 7-10g and h), this combination resulted in a crest width of 7 mm with a dense buccal bone plate (Figs 7-10i and j), allowing the placement of an ITI implant in a good prosthetic position (Figs 7-10k to m). After a tissue integration period of 3 months, the osseointegrated implant was restored with a screw-retained single crown (Figs 7-10n to r).

The use of autogenous bone grafts in combination with barrier membranes was the last major modification of the GBR technique for localized ridge augmentation.

Localized ridge augmentation in a single-tooth gap in area 12 (membrane surgery November 1988).
Figs 7-2a and b

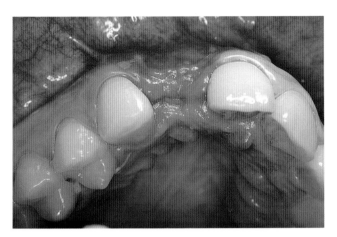

7-2a

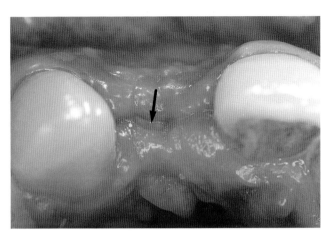

7-2b

Localized ridge augmentation in the left mandible (membrane surgery May 1989).   *Figs 7-3a and b*

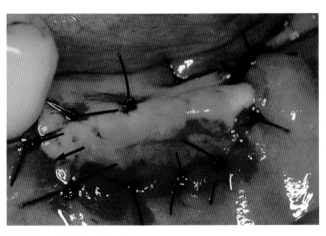

7-3a

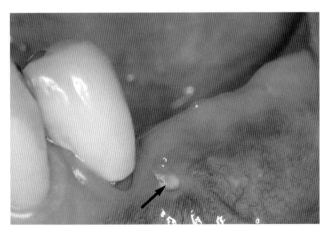

7-3b

Fig 7-2a   Small soft tissue dehiscence 2 months after membrane surgery.

Fig 7-2b   Close-up view of the 2- to 3-mm soft tissue dehiscence *(arrow)*, which later led to an acute infection in the membrane site.

Fig 7-3a   Status following wound closure with an inappropriate vertical relieving incision mesially *(arrow)*.

Fig 7-3b   Soft tissue dehiscence with exposure of the mesial membrane margin in the area of the mesial vertical relieving incision *(arrow)*.

Localized ridge augmentation in a single-tooth gap in area 22 (membrane surgery December 1988).

Figs 7-4a to j

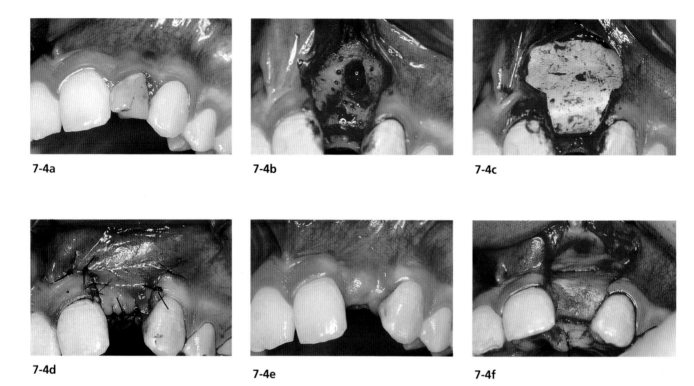

7-4a

7-4b

7-4c

7-4d

7-4e

7-4f

Fig 7-4a Status following complete root resorption of a traumatically injured lateral incisor requiring the extraction of the tooth.

Fig 7-4b Extended bone defect in the alveolar ridge following removal of intraosseous remnants of root canal filling material and granulation tissue.

Fig 7-4c Placement of an e-PTFE membrane (prototype), creating a secluded space in the defect area.

Fig 7-4d Primary wound closure with interrupted single sutures.

Fig 7-4e Status after a complication-free soft tissue healing period of 9 months.

Fig 7-4f Intrasurgical status at reopening with the membrane still in proper position.

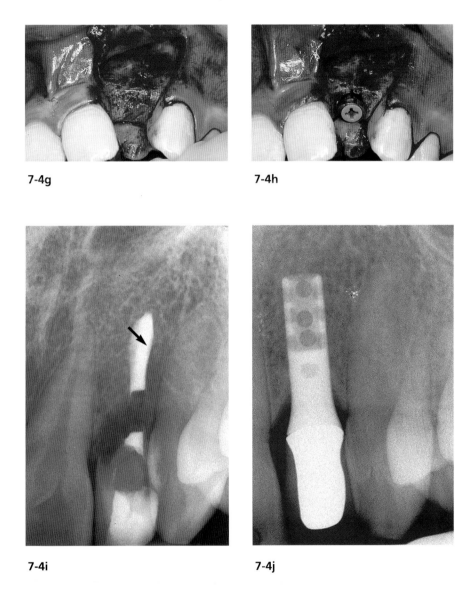

7-4g

7-4h

7-4i

7-4j

Fig 7-4g   Newly augmented ridge with a crest width of more than 7 mm.

Fig 7-4h   Placement of an ITI implant into the newly augmented ridge.

Fig 7-4i   Periapical radiograph at beginning of the treatment shows the remnants of the root canal filling material *(arrow)* and the bone defect in the crestal area.

Fig 7-4j   Periapical radiograph 4 years following implant placement shows regular peri-implant bone structures.

Postoperative complication caused by improper membrane placement (membrane surgery May 1989).
Figs 7-5a to d

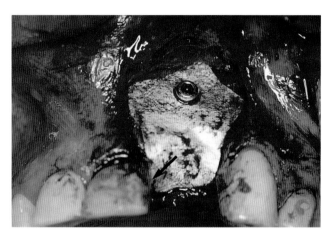

7-5a

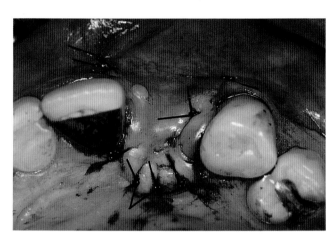

7-5b

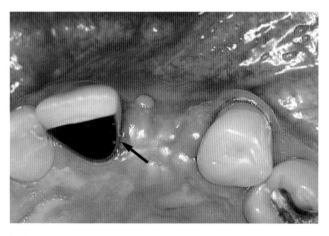

7-5c

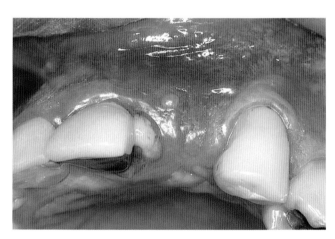

7-5d

Fig 7-5a   Intrasurgical status shows the membrane extending into the sulcus of the adjacent central incisor *(arrow)*.

Fig 7-5b   Wound closure of the membrane site, previously opened with a lateral incision technique on the palatal aspect.

Fig 7-5c   Status 4 weeks after membrane surgery. Note the inflamed soft tissue at the gingival margin of the adjacent central incisor *(arrow)*.

Fig 7-5d   Acute infection 2½ months after membrane surgery in the sulcus of the central incisor.

Specially designed instruments to facilitate membrane placement.
Figs 7-6a to d

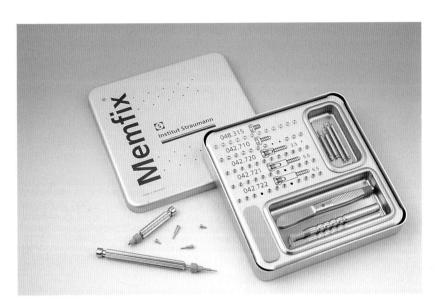

7-6a

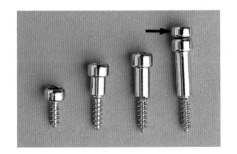

7-6b

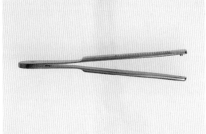

7-6c

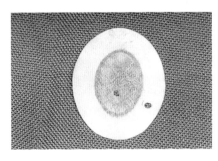

7-6d

Fig 7-6a   Memfix kit containing mini-screws and instruments.

Fig 7-6b   Mini-screws of the Memfix kit. *From left:* Fixation screw; short, medium, and long supporting screws with an inserted head screw *(arrow).*

Fig 7-6c   Membrane punch for cutting small perforations in the membrane for fixation and/or the head screws.

Fig 7-6d   Membrane with two punched holes.

Membrane collapse (membrane surgery April 1989).
Figs 7-7a and b

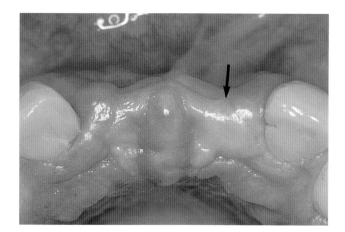

7-7a

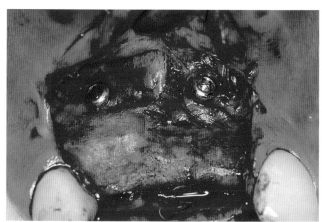

7-7b

Fig 7-7a Clinical status following membrane surgery demonstrates the buccal collapse in the area of the left central incisor *(arrow).*

Fig 7-7b Intrasurgical status at reopening demonstrates the collapse of the membrane in area 21.

Partial membrane collapse (membrane surgery September 1990).
Figs 7-8a to d

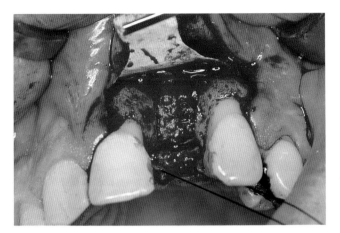

7-8a

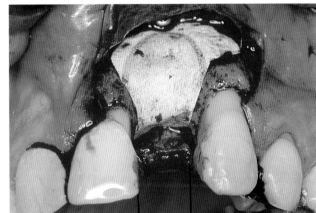

7-8b

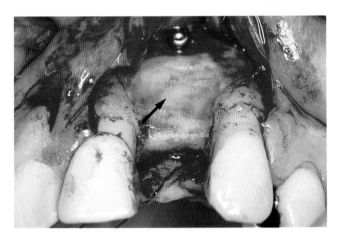

7-8c

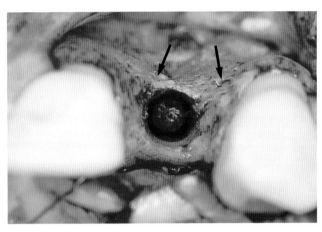

7-8d

Fig 7-8a Defect in the alveolar ridge is filled with a collagen sponge to stabilize the blood clot.

Fig 7-8b Application of e-PTFE membrane and stabilization with a fixation screw.

Fig 7-8c Reopening status 9 months following membrane surgery. Note the partial collapse of the membrane *(arrow)*.

Fig 7-8d Partial collapse of the membrane resulted in a residual facial bone defect *(arrows)*, which caused a slightly more palatal implant site position.

Ridge augmentation in an extended edentulous space in the maxilla (membrane surgery September 1990).

Figs 7-9a to p

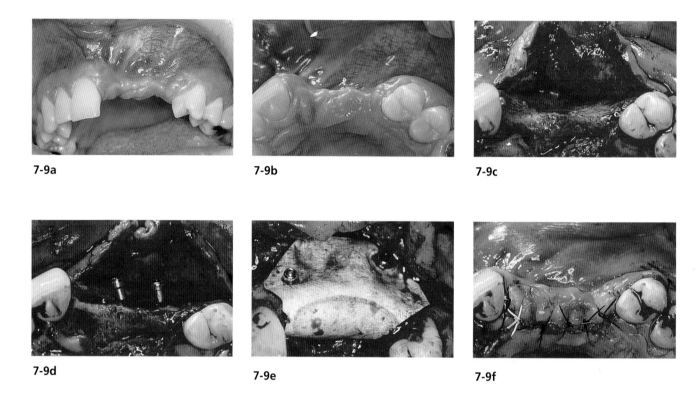

7-9a

7-9b

7-9c

7-9d

7-9e

7-9f

Fig 7-9a   Teeth adjacent to edentulous space (three teeth lost to trauma) are free of fillings and caries.

Fig 7-9b   Occlusal view demonstrates the extended hard and soft tissue defect in the alveolar ridge.

Fig 7-9c   Extended bone defect in the alveolar ridge preventing the placement of dental implants.

Fig 7-9d   Status following placement of two supporting screws as "tent poles" for membrane support.

Fig 7-9e   Placement of a membrane to create a space in the defect area. Membrane stabilization with two fixation screws. The space underneath the membrane was filled with a collagen sponge to stabilize the blood clot.

Fig 7-9f   Primary wound closure with interrupted sutures.

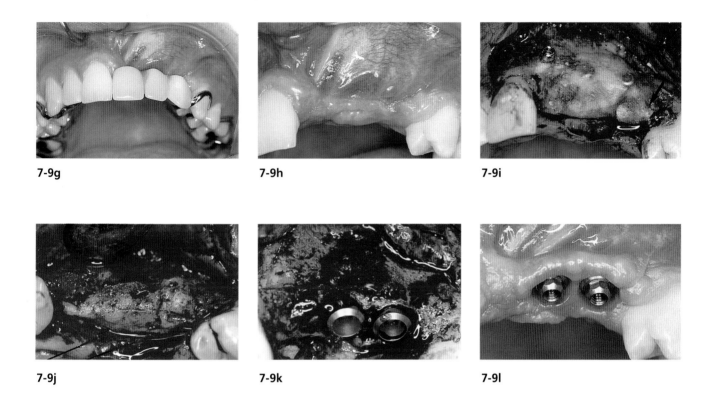

7-9g   7-9h   7-9i

7-9j   7-9k   7-9l

Fig 7-9g Tooth-supported temporary partial denture without direct contact to the soft tissue surface in the membrane site.

Fig 7-9h Clinical status 9 months following membrane surgery and a complication-free wound healing.

Fig 7-9i Intrasurgical status shows the membrane with the fixation screw and two supporting screws appearing through the membrane. Note the partial membrane collapse in area 23/24 *(arrow)*.

Fig 7-9j Occlusal view reveals a sufficient width of 7 mm in area 22/23, allowing the placement of two ITI implants.

Fig 7-9k Placement of two ITI hollow-cylinder implants in area 22/23. Due to the partial membrane collapse, the implants had to be inserted in a more palatal position.

Fig 7-9l Soft tissue status following the tissue integration period and insertion of two Octa-abutments.

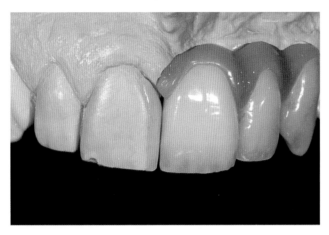

7-9m

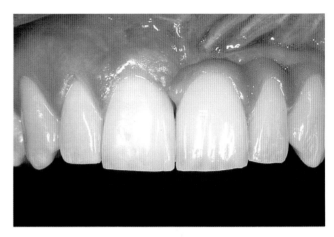

7-9n

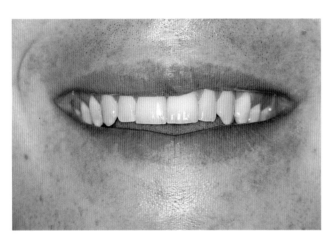

7-9o

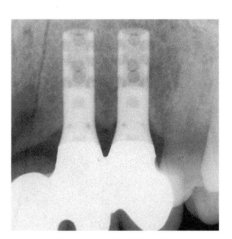

7-9p

Fig 7-9m Master cast with the final restoration of area 21/22/23. To create dimensional harmony, tooth 11 has been enlarged by a mesially located ceramic angle. (Laboratory work: A. Schönenberger, Glattbrugg, Switzerland.)

Fig 7-9n Clinical view of the fixed partial denture with a mesial cantilever unit. Status 2 years following implant insertion. (Prosthetic restoration: Prof Dr U. Belser, University of Geneva, Switzerland.)

Fig 7-9o Final esthetic result.

Fig 7-9p Periapical radiograph with the two hollow-cylinder implants 2 years after implant placement.

Ridge augmentation in a single-tooth gap in area 21 caused by trauma (membrane surgery June 1991).

Figs 7-10a to r

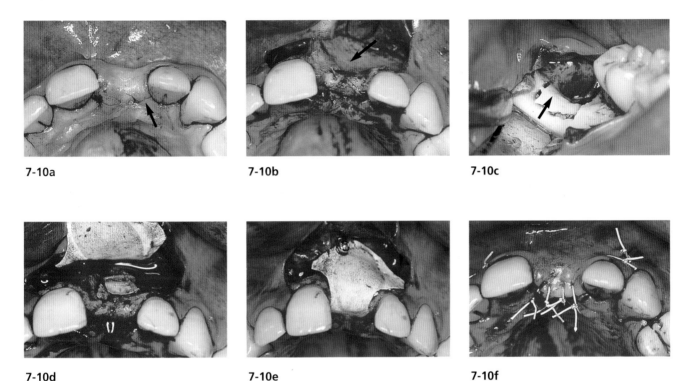

7-10a

7-10b

7-10c

7-10d

7-10e

7-10f

Fig 7-10a   Occlusal view shows the palatal incision *(arrow)* approximately 3 to 4 mm from the midcrest.

Fig 7-10b   Status following flap elevation. Note the narrow alveolar crest of approximately 3 mm and the buccal undercut *(arrow)* preventing the placement of an implant.

Fig 7-10c   Autogenous bone graft is harvested in the third molar site of the right mandible *(arrow)*.

Fig 7-10d   Bone grafts are placed on the buccal aspect to extend the alveolar ridge and to support the membrane.

Fig 7-10e   Precisely trimmed membrane is placed and affixed to the bone with a fixation screw.

Fig 7-10f   Primary wound closure with interrupted sutures.

Fig 7-10g   Clinical status during the complication-free healing period of 9 months demonstrates the provisional partial denture.

Fig 7-10h   Clinical status 9 months after membrane surgery.

Fig 7-10i   Intrasurgical status at reopening, with the membrane still in proper position.

Fig 7-10j   Occlusal view demonstrates the newly formed crest (7 mm wide) with a dense cortical bone plate at the buccal aspect *(arrow)*.

Fig 7-10k   Preparation of the recipient site for an ITI hollow-cylinder implant. Note the intact central bone core before removal for histologic examination.

Fig 7-10l   Placement of an ITI implant in a good prosthetic position and excellent primary stability. Insertion of a transgingival healing cap.

Fig 7-10m   Close adaptation of the wound margin to the healing cap, and wound closure with interrupted sutures.

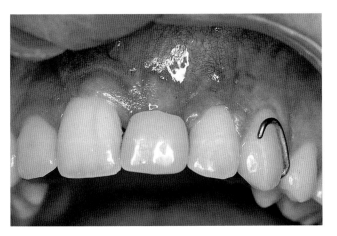

7-10g

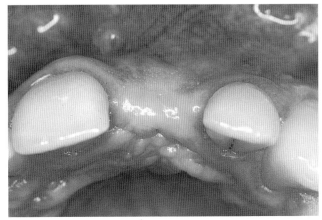

7-10h

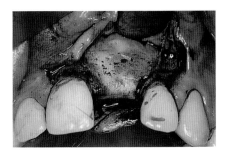

7-10i

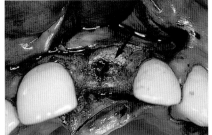

7-10j

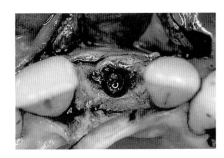

7-10k

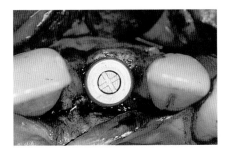

7-10l

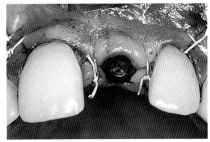

7-10m

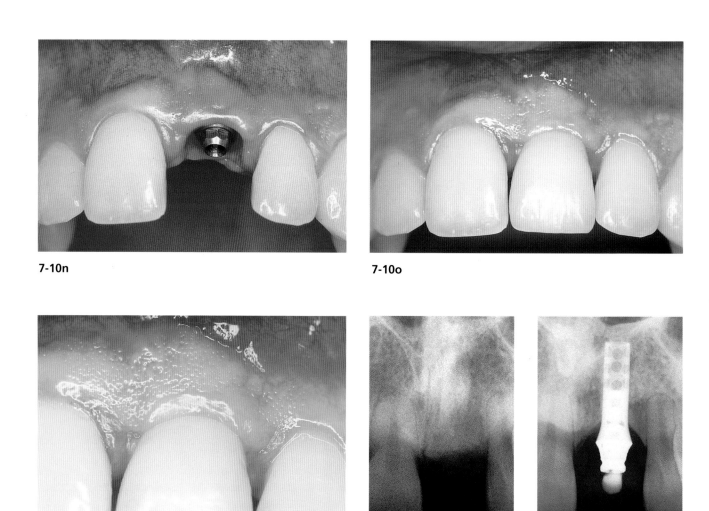

7-10n

7-10o

7-10p

7-10q

7-10r

Fig 7-10n Status following the healing period of 3 months and insertion of an Octa-abutment for a screw-retained crown.

Fig 7-10o Provisional restoration with a screw-retained acrylic resin crown mounted to a precisely fitting gold coping. (Prosthetic restoration: Dr J.-P. Martinet, University of Geneva, Switzerland).

Fig 7-10p Detailed view demonstrates the nice gingival contour of the peri-implant soft tissues without clinical signs of inflammation.

Fig 7-10q Preoperative radiograph shows the single-tooth gap and signs of root resorption at the neighboring teeth.

Fig 7-10r Radiograph 7 months after implant placement reveals the osseointegrated implant with normal bone structures.

Current Surgical Technique

Based on the learning experience from 1988 to 1991, the following surgical technique for localized ridge augmentation is routinely used at the Department of Oral Surgery, University of Berne. The technique for localized ridge augmentation in the mandible and in the maxilla are presented in detail.

Surgical Infrastructure and Preoperative Preparation

In general, GBR procedures are carried out in an operating room under strict hygienic conditions. This includes a preoperative mouthwash of the patient's oral cavity with chlorhexidine digluconate 0.2% (1 minute) and perioral skin disinfection. Patients are covered with sterile sheets to minimize contamination of the wound with extraoral bacteria (Fig 7-11a). The surgeon and the assistants wear face masks, caps, protection glasses, sterile surgical gowns, and sterile gloves (Fig 7-11b). The surgeries are performed with local anesthesia (5 to 10 mL articaine 4% with epinephrine 1:100,000) combined with a sedative (5 mg Midazolam intramuscularly) and an antisialagogue (0.5 mg atropine intramuscularly) premedication. Furthermore, patients are given a perioperative antibiotic prophylaxis for 2 to 3 days (amoxicillin 750 mg orally 2 hours preoperatively and every 6 hours postoperatively). The surgical procedure is performed with a standard instrument set for implant and membrane surgeries (Fig 7-11c) that includes especially fine instruments (Implant and Membrane Surgical Kit, Hu-Friedy, Chicago, IL) to allow careful and meticulous soft tissue handling (Fig 7-11d).

Surgical Procedure in the Mandible

The step-by-step procedure for ridge augmentation in the mandible is demonstrated in a patient with a distal extension situation exhibiting a narrow alveolar ridge (Figs 7-12a and b). Following local anesthesia, the intact soft tissue cover was opened using a split-thickness incision of the alveolar mucosa carried out on the buccal aspect approximately 3 to 5 mm lateral to the mucogingival junction (Figs 7-12c and d). The flap was extended into the retromolar area to harvest a corticocancellous bone graft. Following epiperiosteal preparation, the periosteum was cut at the level of the mucogingival junction (Fig 7-12e). At the mesial aspect of the flap, the incision was extended into the sulcus of the most distal tooth in the arch. Distally, a divergent full-thickness relieving incision was extended to the lingual aspect. Subsequently, the combined split-thickness/full-thickness flap was carefully elevated with a fine periosteal elevator to the lingual aspect, and the flap was held away with retraction sutures (Fig 7-12f) attached to hemostats. Surgical retractors were not used inside the flap to minimize trauma to the flap. The intrasurgical status confirmed the presence of a narrow alveolar ridge with an insufficient crest width to allow the placement of ITI implants. Remnants of an intraosseous amalgam filling were carefully removed with a round bur. In addition, remnants of the periosteum were completely removed from the bone surface with a surgical curette. Subsequently, a corticocancellous bone graft was harvested from the retromolar area (Fig 7-12g) and a hole was drilled into the graft to allow its fixation to the bone recipient site with a Memfix supporting screw (Fig 7-12h). The graft recipient site was selected, the screw hole for the supporting screw was prepared using the smallest (2.2 mm) pilot drill of the ITI solid-screw instrument kit. The cortical bone surface was perforated to open the marrow space and to achieve a bleeding bone surface. Subsequently, the bone graft was placed and stabilized with a supporting screw (Figs 7-12i and j). The graft was placed with the cortical surface facing buccally, and the cancellous portion in close contact to host bone.

A sterile e-PTFE membrane (GTAM Oval-9) was trimmed with scissors. The membrane was appropriately shaped to extend 3 to 4 mm beyond the defect margins and allow a close adaptation of the membrane to the surrounding bone. Two locations for fixation screws were selected, and small holes were punched into the membrane with the special membrane punch. The membrane was applied to the surgical site and affixed to the bone with two fixation screws on the buccal aspect. The remaining space around the bone graft was filled with bone chips harvested from the retromolar area with a chisel. A long cut was made into the membrane to allow the overlapping of the membrane and close adaptation to the curve of the mandibular arch on the lingual aspect (Figs 7-12k and l). Furthermore, the membrane was precisely trimmed with a scalpel close to the adjacent tooth mesially to create a small zone of uncovered bone for flap attachment and to minimize the risk of membrane contamination from the sulcus. These procedures resulted in the membrane being absolutely stable in situ. Subsequently, wound closure was initiated with three vertical mattress sutures to lift the buccal flap as much as possible (Figs 7-12m and n). With this flap technique, the well-vascularized buccal flap was used to cover the membrane from the lateral aspect, providing a good wound bed for the overlapping lingual flap. These mattress sutures were also used to take up the tension caused by the postoperative swelling. Close adaptation of the wound margins was achieved by numerous interrupted sutures (Figs 7-12o and p).

The patient was instructed not to chew or brush in the treated area for approximately 2 weeks. Chemical plaque control with chlorhexidinedigluconate solution (0.1%, 1 minute tid) was instituted for the first postoperative week. The patient was given a nonsteroidal anti-inflammatory medication (diclofenac 50 mg tid for 3 days) and was instructed to use a cold pack for frequent extraoral application in the surgical area during the first 3 postsurgical days. A tight extraoral elastoplast pressure dressing was applied to minimize the postoperative swelling in the wound area. The antibiotic prophylaxis was given as outlined above. Furthermore, the patient was asked to apply Solcoseryl dental adhesive paste (Solco Basel, Birsfelden, Switzerland) to the surgical site with cotton swabs three times per day for approximately 3 weeks (Fig 7-12q). This paste fosters soft tissue healing by granulation and contains an analgesic component for local pain relief. Because of the extended surgical site with lack of a distal tooth, the patient was instructed not to wear a temporary partial denture during the healing period to avoid direct pressure to the membrane site.

The patient was recalled 2 and 7 days following surgery. At 7 days, the interrupted sutures were carefully removed following careful cleansing of the wound. For the second and third weeks following surgery, the chlorhexidine mouthwash was replaced by a chlorhexidine gel (Plak Out gel 0.2%, Hawe Neos AG, Gentilino, Switzerland) which the patient applied to the site with cotton swabs three times daily. The vertical mattress sutures were removed after 14 days of healing (Fig 7-12r). Subsequently, the patient was seen once a week until the primary soft tissue healing was completed. After this, the patient was recalled every 4 weeks to examine the soft tissue status. Nine months after membrane surgery, clinical examination demonstrated asymptomatic healing and no soft tissue dehiscence with membrane exposure (Fig 7-12s). The site was reopened with a crestal incision (Fig 7-12t), and the membrane was removed. The intrasurgical status demonstrated a crest width of approximately 8 mm, allowing the placement of three ITI implants in appropriate implant positions with excellent primary stability (Figs 7-12u to w). After the placement of healing caps, the wound margins were carefully adapted and secured in position with interrupted sutures (Fig 7-12x). Finally, the inserted implants demonstrated an uneventful tissue integration. After 3 months of healing, the implants were ankylotically stable and showed no evidence of soft tissue inflammation (Fig 7-13a). Thus, the prosthetic abutments were inserted (Fig 7-13b) and the patient was restored as part of a comprehensive treatment with a five-unit cantilever fixed partial denture (Figs 7-13c to f).

Surgical Procedure in the Maxilla

The surgical procedure in the maxilla has some specific differences, but the basic surgical technique is the same as that for the mandible. The step-by-step procedure is presented in a patient exhibiting an extended edentulous space in the left maxilla with four missing teeth (Fig 7-14a). Contrary to the technique in the mandible, the lateral split-thickness incision of the mucosa was made on the palatal aspect (Figs 7-14b and c). Mesially, the incision was extended through the sulcus of tooth 22 to the buccal aspect and relieved into the vestibule with a vertical distal line angle full-thickness incision. Distally, a divergent full-thickness relieving incision was made in the area of the first molar. Following supra-periosteal preparation of the buccal flap, the periosteum was cut and the combined split-thickness/full-thickness flap could be elevated with a fine periosteal elevator. Flap handling and debridement of the bone surface were carried out as described previously. The intrasurgical status confirmed the narrow alveolar ridge and the need for ridge augmentation (Fig 7-14d). Subsequently, a corticocancellous bone graft was harvested in the chin area and applied to the buccal aspect in area 23/24 (Fig 7-14e). The graft was stabilized with a supporting screw. A sterile e-PTFE membrane (GTAM Oval-9) was trimmed with scissors and appropriately shaped to extend 3 to 4 mm beyond the defect margins. The membrane was applied to the surgical site and affixed to the bone with two fixation screws at the buccal aspect (Fig 7-14f). With this fixation, the membrane was absolutely stable in situ. Prior to wound closure, the periosteum of the buccal flap was carefully relieved to achieve a tension-free adaptation of the wound margins. Subsequently, wound closure was initiated with three horizontal mattress sutures and completed with numerous interrupted sutures (Fig 7-14g).

The postoperative medication was the same as described for the previous patient. The examination 7 days after surgery demonstrated a superficial necrosis of the epithelium at the tip of the buccal flap (Fig 7-14h), which is frequently seen in the maxilla. To accelerate the concentric re-epithelization, dental adhesive paste was applied by the patient 3 times daily with cotton swabs. The interrupted single sutures were removed after 7 days, whereas the mattress sutures remained in place for another week of healing. Approximately 4 weeks after surgery the soft tissue healing was completed, and the patient was recalled every 4 weeks for examination. The site was reopened after 9 months of complication-free soft tissue healing (Fig 7-14i). Following removal of the membrane, the intrasurgical status demonstrated a crest width of 6 to 7 mm, allowing the placement of two ITI implants in area 23/24 (Fig 7-14j to l). The implants were placed deeper in the bone than usual for esthetic reasons. Following insertion of transgingival healing caps to extend the implant to the soft tissue surface, the peri-implant mucosa was carefully adapted to the healing caps and secured in position with interrupted sutures to permit nonsubmerged healing of these implants (Fig 7-14m). After a complication-free tissue integration period of 3 months (Fig 7-14n to p), the implants were restored with a combined tooth/implant-supported five-unit fixed partial denture.

The current surgical technique carried out in another patient with a single-tooth gap in the maxilla is demonstrated in Figs 7-15a to r.

Surgical protocol and instrumentation.
Figs 7-11a to d

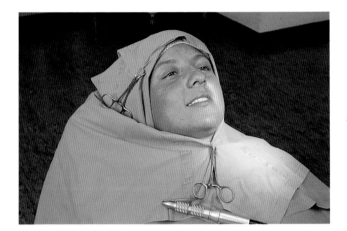

7-11a

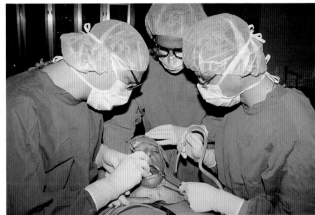

7-11b

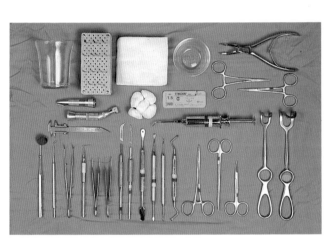

7-11c

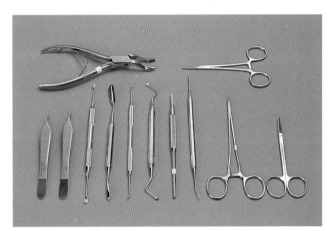

7-11d

Fig 7-11a Perioral skin disinfection and coverage of the patient with sterile sheets to minimize the risk of bacterial wound contamination during the surgical procedure.

Fig 7-11b Surgeon and the two assistants wear sterile gowns, face masks, caps, protective glasses, and gloves during membrane surgery.

Fig 7-11c Surgical instrument kit for membrane surgery.

Fig 7-11d Specially designed instruments (Hu-Friedy) for low-trauma soft tissue handling and precise membrane placement.

Fig 7-12a   Occlusal view shows the clinical status in the mandible at the beginning of a complete comprehensive treatment.

Fig 7-12b   Lateral view of the distal extension situation of the right mandible with an insufficient crest width for implant placement.

Fig 7-12c   Split-thickness incision of the mucosa at the buccal aspect. Extension of the incision into the retromolar area for bone graft harvesting.

Fig 7-12d   Schematic drawing of the lateral incision technique on the buccal aspect with a supraperiosteal preparation for a combined split- and full-thickness flap.

Fig 7-12e   Incision of the periosteum at the height of the mucogingival junction. The buccal flap is already partially elevated *(arrows)*.

Fig 7-12f   Elevation of the flap to the lingual aspect. The flap is gently held in place with retraction suture *(arrow)*.

Ridge augmentation in a distal extension situation in the mandible (membrane surgery March 1992).

Figs 7-12a to 13f

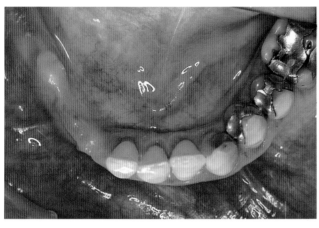

7-12a

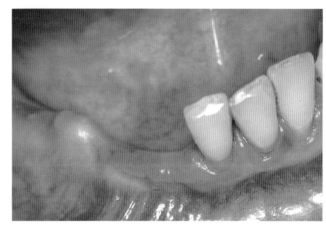

7-12b

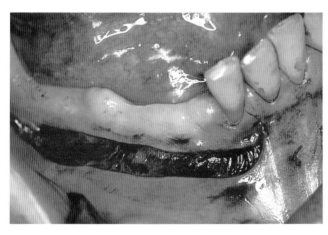

7-12c

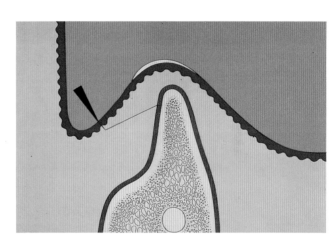

7-12d

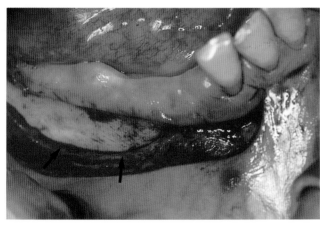

7-12e

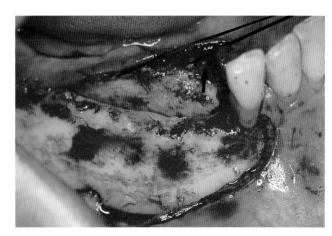

7-12f

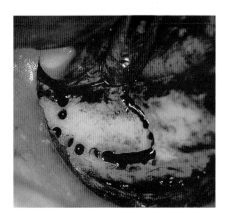

7-12g

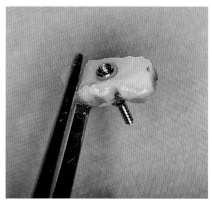

7-12h

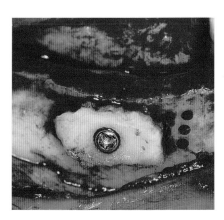

7-12i

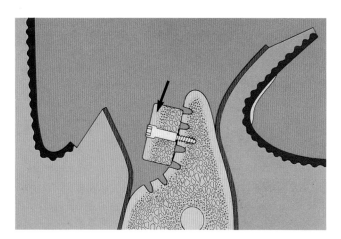

7-12j

Fig 7-12g Harvesting of a corticocancellous bone graft in the retromolar area within the limits of the same flap.

Fig 7-12h Perforation of the bone graft for a supporting screw.

Fig 7-12i Placement of the corticocancellous bone graft lateral to the alveolar crest. Stabilization of the graft with a supporting screw.

Fig 7-12j Schematic diagram of graft application. The cancellous portion of the graft is in close contact with the local bone, whereas the cortical layer *(arrow)* is facing buccally.

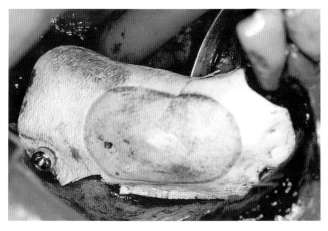

7-12k

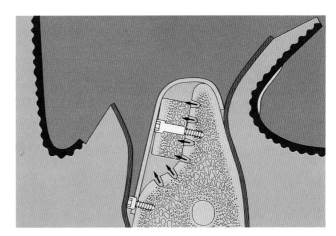

7-12l

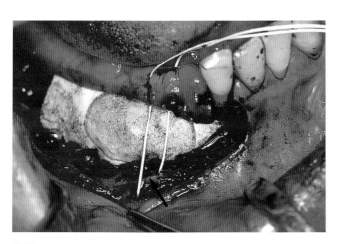

7-12m

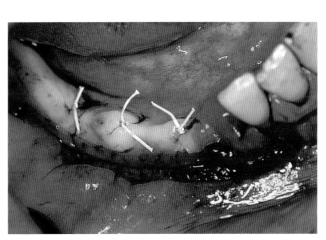

7-12n

Fig 7-12k   Placement of a trimmed e-PTFE membrane (GTAM Oval-9) to cover the defect and the bone graft. The membrane is stabilized with two fixation screws at the buccal aspect and tucked underneath the mucoperiosteal flap lingually.

Fig 7-12l   Schematic diagram of membrane application. Note the numerous perforations in the cortical bone, allowing the migration of angiogenic and osteogenic cells into the secluded space *(arrows)*.

Fig 7-12m   Initiation of wound closure with vertical mattress sutures. The sutures pick up the buccal flap going deep through the supraperiosteal connective tissue *(arrow)*.

Fig 7-12n   Status following closure with the three mattress sutures. To avoid flap necrosis, the sutures should not be tightened too much.

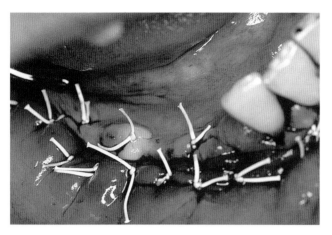

7-12o

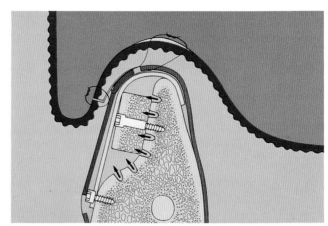

7-12p

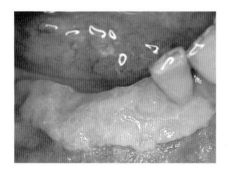

7-12q

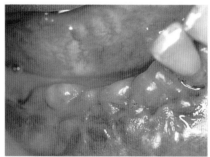

7-12r

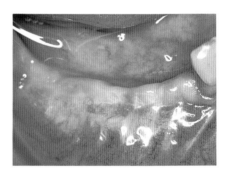

7-12s

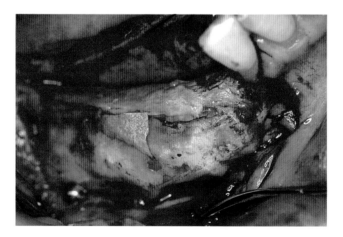

7-12t

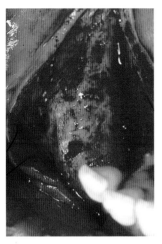
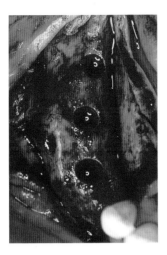
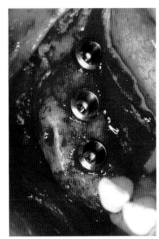
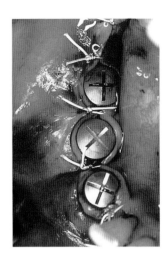

7-12u   7-12v   7-12w   7-12x

Fig 7-12o Completion of wound closure with numerous interrupted sutures at the buccal incision.

Fig 7-12p Schematic diagram of the suturing technique.

Fig 7-12q Wound dressing with frequent application of Solcoseryl dental adhesive paste to accelerate soft tissue healing.

Fig 7-12r Clinical status 14 days following membrane surgery and suture removal.

Fig 7-12s Status 9 months following a complication-free soft tissue healing.

Fig 7-12t Intrasurgical status at reopening, with the membrane still in place.

Fig 7-12u Occlusal view of the newly formed alveolar ridge. The width of the crest measures approximately 8 mm in area 43/44/45.

Fig 7-12v Occlusal view after preparation of the recipient sites for three ITI implants.

Fig 7-12w Occlusal view after insertion of three ITI implants into the newly augmented alveolar ridge. Note the thick buccal bone wall on implants 43 and 44/45.

Fig 7-12x Occlusal view after application of healing caps and wound closure with interrupted sutures.

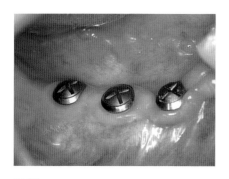

7-13a

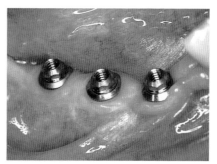

7-13b

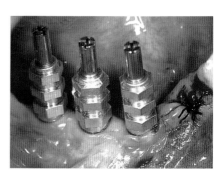

7-13c

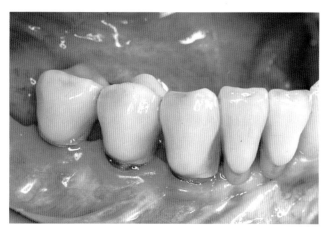

7-13d

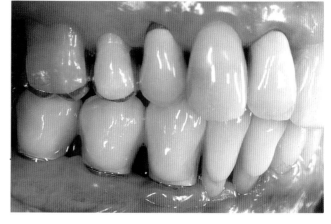

7-13e

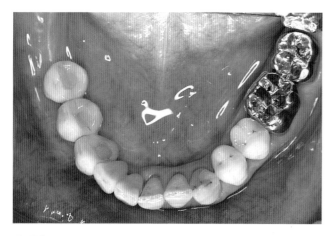

7-13f

Fig 7-13a   Clinical status 3 months after implant placement.

Fig 7-13b   Status following insertion of three Octa-abutments.

Fig 7-13c   Placement of transfer copings of the Octa system for precise transfer. The mandibular incisor has been extracted for periodontal reasons.

Fig 7-13d   Lateral view of the implant-supported five-unit fixed partial denture with two mesial cantilever units. (Prosthetic restoration by Dr B. Hugo, University of Berne; laboratory work by Mr B. Heckendorn, Labor Busch, Bern, Switzerland.)

Fig 7-13e   Lateral view of the implant-supported restoration in occlusion with the opposing maxilla.

Fig 7-13f   Occlusal view of the mandible following completion of comprehensive treatment.

Localized ridge augmentation in the left maxilla (membrane surgery February 1992). *Figs 7-14a to p*

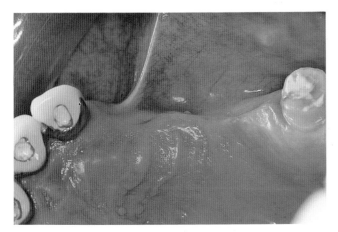

7-14a

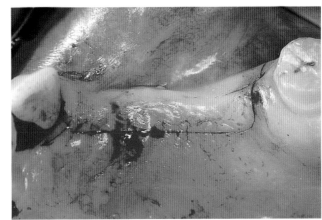

7-14b

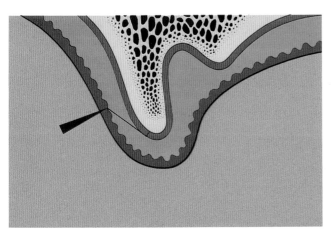

7-14c

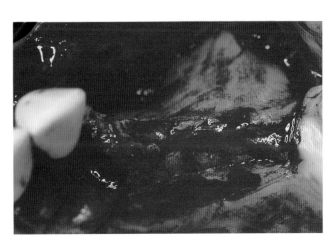

7-14d

Fig 7-14a   Extended edentulous space; status following surgical removal of a horizontally impacted canine.

Fig 7-14b   Lateral incision technique at the palatal aspect of the ridge with a split-thickness incision of the mucosa.

Fig 7-14c   Schematic diagram of the incision technique in the maxilla. Note the supraperiosteal preparation of the flap to extend the wound surface at the incision line.

Fig 7-14d   Status following flap elevation. The alveolar crest demonstrates an insufficient width for implant placement.

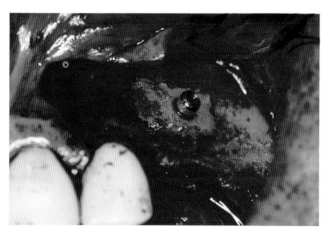

7-14e

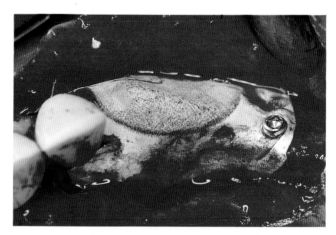

7-14f

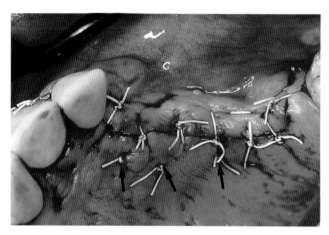

7-14g

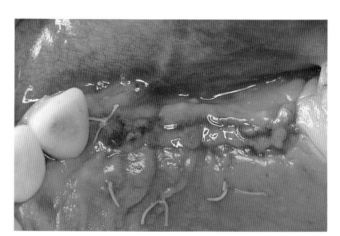

7-14h

Fig 7-14e Application of a corticocancellous bone graft for lateral ridge augmentation. The graft is stabilized with a supporting screw.

Fig 7-14f Application of a membrane to create a space, and membrane stabilization with two fixation screws.

Fig 7-14g Primary wound closure with three mattress sutures *(arrows)* and interrupted sutures.

Fig 7-14h Clinical status 7 days after surgery. The intact connective tissue heals by granulation due to a superficial necrosis of the epithelial layer. The mattress sutures are left in place for a second week.

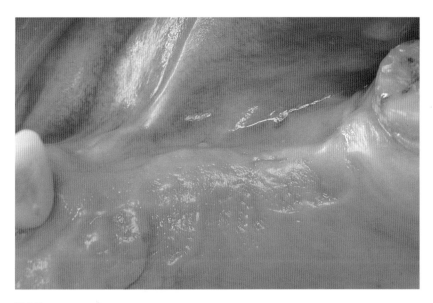

7-14i

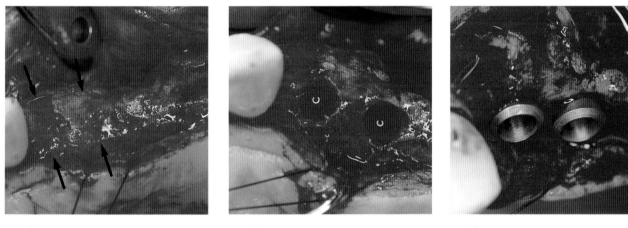

7-14j   7-14k   7-14l

Fig 7-14i Clinical status after complication-free wound healing of 9 months.

Fig 7-14j Clinical status at reopening and following membrane removal. Note the enlarged alveolar crest in area 23/24 *(arrows)*.

Fig 7-14k Preparation of two recipient sites for ITI implants. Note the thick buccal bone wall in area 23.

Fig 7-14l Insertion of two ITI screw implants.

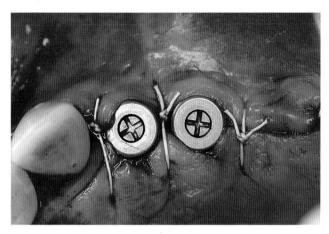

7-14m

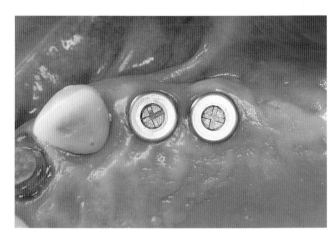

7-14n

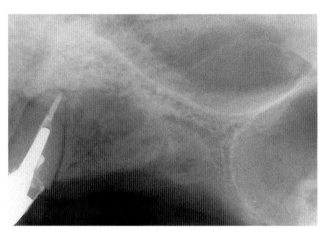

7-14o

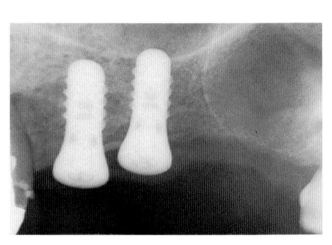

7-14p

Fig 7-14m Clinical status following placement of transgingival healing caps, close adaptation of the wound margins, and wound closure with interrupted sutures.

Fig 7-14n Status 3 months after implant placement. The implants achieved a successful tissue integration with ankylotic stability.

Fig 7-14o Radiographic status at the beginning of the treatment with an extended bone defect in area 23/24 caused by the surgically removed impacted canine.

Fig 7-14p Radiograph at the end of the 3-month tissue integration period shows regular peri-implant bone structures.

Localized ridge augmentation in a single-tooth gap (membrane surgery July 1992). *Figs 7-15a to r*

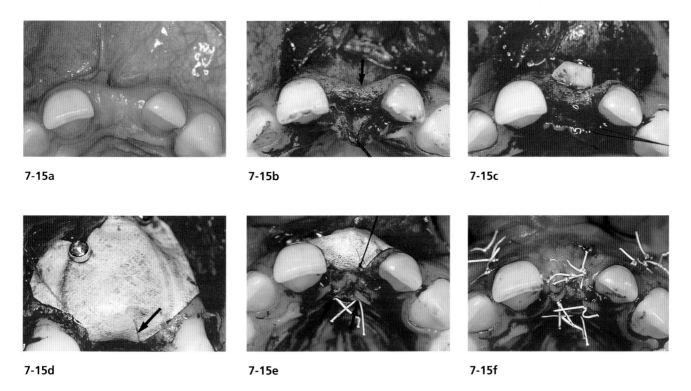

7-15a

7-15b

7-15c

7-15d

7-15e

7-15f

Fig 7-15a Occlusal view reveals the collapse of the alveolar crest in area 21.

Fig 7-15b Intrasurgical status. The narrow alveolar crest is caused by the buccal atrophy *(arrow)*, preventing the placement of an implant.

Fig 7-15c Application of an autogenous corticocancellous bone graft to enlarge the ridge width. Stabilization of the graft is achieved with a supporting screw of the Memfix kit.

Fig 7-15d Application of an e-PTFE membrane to create a space to cover the bone graft. Membrane is stabilized with two fixation screws. Note the cut in the membrane *(arrow)* for an overlapping membrane adaptation in the crest area.

Fig 7-15e Occlusal view demonstrates the close adaptation of the membrane to the palate. The membrane is pulled to the palate by two vertical mattress sutures *(arrows)*.

Fig 7-15f Primary wound closure with mattress and interrupted sutures.

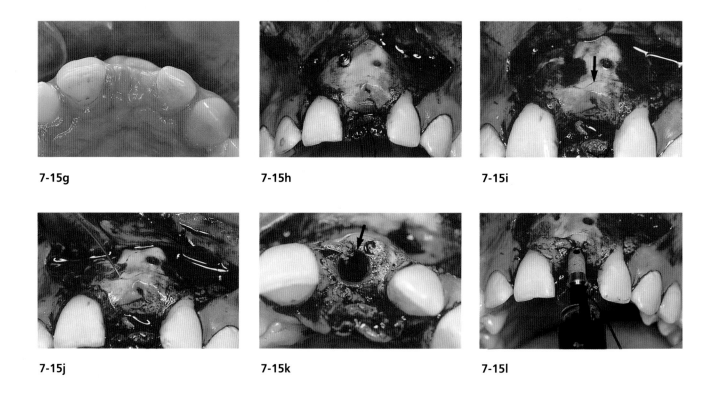

7-15g

7-15h

7-15i

7-15j

7-15k

7-15l

Fig 7-15g Clinical status at the end of a complication-free healing period of 9 months.

Fig 7-15h Intrasurgical status at reopening. The membrane is still in proper position.

Fig 7-15i Status following membrane removal. A thin soft tissue layer is found underneath the membrane *(arrow)*.

Fig 7-15j Thin soft tissue layer is probed with a fine needle to examine the thickness. This layer is left in place at the buccal aspect.

Fig 7-15k Preparation of a recipient site for an ITI hollow-cylinder implant in an appropriate position from a prosthetic point of view. Note the thick buccal bone wall *(arrow)*.

Fig 7-15l Insertion of an angled hollow-cylinder implant to achieve a correct implant axis.

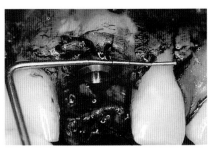

7-15m

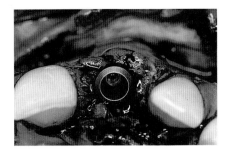

7-15n

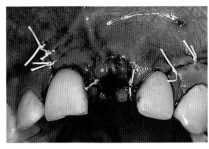

7-15o

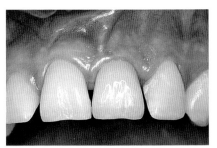

7-15p

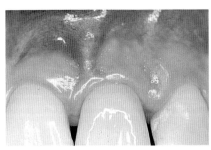

7-15q

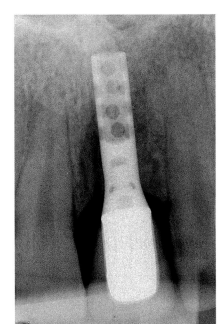

7-15r

Fig 7-15m   Implant shoulder is located approximately 1 mm above the alveolar crest and slightly below the cementoenamel junction of the adjacent teeth.

Fig 7-15n   Occlusal view demonstrates the correct orofacial position of the implant for an esthetic implant restoration.

Fig 7-15o   Adaptation of the wound margins and closure with interrupted sutures. Note the buccal wound margin placed on top of the healing cap and the correct position of the papillae.

Fig 7-15p   Clinical status after restoration of the implant with a screw-retained metal-ceramic crown demonstrating a pleasing esthetic result with harmonious gingival contours. (Prosthetic restoration by Dr D. Hess, University of Berne; laboratory work by Mr B. Heckendorn, Labor Busch, Bern, Switzerland.)

Fig 7-15q   Close-up view demonstrates the clinically healthy peri-implant soft tissues.

Fig 7-15r   Periapical radiograph 6 months after implant placement demonstrates the restored ITI hollow-cylinder implant with normal peri-implant bone structures.

Results From 1988 to 1993

Between November 1988 and January 1993, a total of 40 patients were consecutively treated with the GBR technique for localized ridge augmentation and admitted to a clinical study. To demonstrate the development of the presented surgical technique, the patients were divided into three groups according to treatment date (Fig 7-16). Table 1 provides detailed information about each patient, including indication and location, dates of surgeries, surgical technique, postoperative complications, number of implants placed, as well as the overall result.

The collected clinical data of the patients in group 1 have already been published.[1] In this group the main complication was flap dehiscence, observed in five patients. Three of them developed acute infection in the membrane site within 3 months of membrane placement. This soft tissue complication required membrane removal, and the three patients with acute infection demonstrated insufficient crest width that prevented the placement of dental implants. As mentioned previously, another patient demonstrated complete membrane collapse that resulted in an insufficient crest width for implant placement. Analysis of the results of group 1 demonstrates significant complications in six patients (50%); only 8 of 12 patients (66%) received implants.

With more clinical experience and the development of a modified, enhanced surgical technique, the rate of complications was significantly reduced in groups 2 and 3. Only 1 of 28 patients (<4%) exhibited flap dehiscence with membrane exposure. An acute infection was avoided because the membrane was partially removed after 2 months of healing. Partial membrane collapse was observed in a few patients. In two patients, an implant could not be inserted, resulting in a negative outcome of the procedure. One patient demonstrated scar tissue formation underneath the membrane, possibly due to insufficient debridement of the exist-

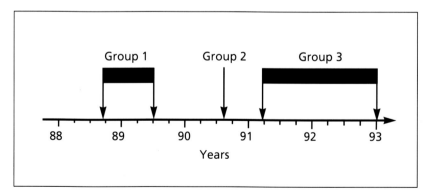

Fig 7-16 Treatment timetable: Patients treated with localized ridge augmentation using GBR.

Table 7-1 *Indications, Postoperative Complications, and Results of 40 Patients Treated With the GBR Technique for Localized Ridge Augmentation (Nov 88–Jan 93)*

Patient no.	Indication	Membrane surgery		Complications	Second surgery	Site implants placed	Result
		Date	Materials used				
Group 1							
1	Single-tooth gap 12	Nov 88	GTAM & Collagen	Flap dehiscence & infection	–	None	–
2	Single-tooth gap 22	Dec 88	GTAM & Collagen	–	Oct 89	22	++
3	Single-tooth gap 22	Apr 89	GTAM & Collagen	–	Jan 90	22	++
4	Single-tooth gap 21	May 89	GTAM & Collagen	Infection in sulcus 11	–	None	–
5	Edentulous space 11/21	May 89	GTAM & Collagen	Complete membrane collapse	Jan 90	None	–
6	Single-tooth gap 12	May 89	GTAM & Collagen	Flap dehiscence & infection	–	None	–
7	Edentulous space 13-11	May 89	GTAM & Collagen	–	Jan 90	12, 13	++
8	Edentulous space 34-37	Jun 89	GTAM & Collagen	–	Apr 90	34, 36	++
9	Distal extension 36	Jul 89	GTAM & Collagen	–	Apr 90	36	++
10	Single-tooth gap 14	Jul 89	GTAM & Collagen	Flap dehiscence w/o infection	Feb 90	14	++
11	Distal extension 34-36	Jul 89	GTAM & Collagen	Flap dehiscence w/o infection	Apr 90	34, 36	++
12	Single-tooth gap 46	Jul 89	GTAM & Collagen	–	Apr 90	46	++
Group 2							
13	Edentulous space 21-23	Sep 90	GTAM & Collagen	Partial membrane collapse	Jun 91	22, 23	++
14	Edentulous space 21/22	Sep 90	GTAM & Collagen	–	May 91	None	–
15	Edentulous space 12-22	Sep 90	GTAM & Collagen	–	May 91	12, 22	++
16	Single-tooth gap 22	Sep 90	GTAM & Collagen	Partial membrane collapse	May 91	22	++
17	Single-tooth gap 11	Sep 90	GTAM & Collagen	–	May 91	11*	+
18	Distal extension 14/15	Sep 90	GTAM & Collagen	–	May 91	14, 15*	+
19	Single-tooth gap 11	Sep 90	GTAM & Collagen	Partial membrane collapse	May 91	11**	+
20	Edentulous space 11/21	Sep 90	GTAM & Collagen	–	Jun 91	11, 21	++
21	Single-tooth gap 21	Sep 90	GTAM & Collagen	–	May 91	21	++
Group 3							
22	Distal extension 14-16	Apr 91	GTAM & Collagen	–	Mar 92	13*, 14*, 15*	+
23	Distal extension 45-47	May 91	GTAM & Collagen	Partial membrane collapse	May 92	None	–
24	Single-tooth gap 22	May 91	GTAM & Collagen	–	Feb 92	22	++
25	Edentulous space 21/22	May 91	GTAM & Bone grafts	–	Mar 92	21, 22	++
26	Single-tooth gap 21	Jun 91	GTAM & Bone grafts	–	Mar 92	21	++
27	Edentulous space 45/46	Jun 91	GTAM & Bone grafts	–	May 92	45*, 46	++
28	Edentulous space 23-26	Aug 91	GTAM & Bone grafts	–	May 92	23, 24	++
29	Distal extension 23-26	Aug 91	GTAM & Bone grafts	–	Oct 92	23, 24*	++
30	Single-tooth gap 41	Sep 91	GTAM & Bone grafts	–	May 92	41*	++
31	Edentulous space 11/21	Dec 91	GTAM & Bone grafts	–	Oct 92	11, 21	++
32	Single-tooth gap 21	Dec 91	GTAM & Bone grafts	Flap dehiscence w/o infection	Jan 93	21	++
33	Edentulous space 23-26	Feb 92	GTAM & Bone grafts	–	Oct 92	23, 24	++
34	Distal extension 43-46	Mar 92	GTAM & Bone grafts	–	Dec 92	43, 44/45, 46	++
35	Edentulous space 21/22	May 92	GTAM & Bone grafts	–	Jun 93	21*, 22*	+
36	Distal extension 24-26	Jul 92	GTAM & Bone grafts	–	Apr 93	24, 25	++
37	Single-tooth gap 21	Jul 92	GTAM & Bone grafts	–	May 93	21	++
38	Distal extension 24/25	Jul 92	GTAM & Bone grafts	–	May 93	25*, 26	++/+
39	Distal extension 45/46	Nov 92	GTAM & Bone grafts	–	Sep 93	45, 46	++
40	Distal extension 44-46	Jan 93	GTAM & Bone grafts	–	Oct 93	44, 45, 46*	++/+

Tooth numbering according to WHO; *reduced-diameter ITI implant could be inserted (ø 3.3 mm); **implant was inserted with simultaneous membrane placement.
 –Failure, no implant placement.
 +Successful ridge augmentation for the placement of reduced-diameter ITI implants.
 ++Successful ridge augmentation for the placement of standard ITI implants.

ing infrabony defect during the first surgery. In the other patient the attempt for vertical ridge augmentation in a distal extension situation in the mandible was not successful. Since the decision to use autogenous bone grafts in combination with e-PTFE membranes, membrane collapse has not been observed and all patients have demonstrated successful results with the GBR technique for localized ridge augmentation (ie, ITI implants could be inserted into the newly augmented ridge in all patients).

A direct comparison of the clinical results of group 1 with those of groups 2 and 3 together indicates that the rate of complications with flap dehiscences was reduced from 41% to 4% and the success rate was improved from 66% to 92%.

Keys to Achieving Predictable Results

The goal of the staged approach for guided bone regeneration is, initially, localized ridge augmentation, with subsequent placement of endosseous implants into the newly augmented alveolar ridge following a healing period of 9 months. As described in this chapter, this surgical technique was incrementally modified during a period of 3 years to improve the predictability of the procedure. Clinical results after this period of development indicate that the predictability of the GBR technique for localized ridge augmentation can be improved when the surgical technique is followed and certain goals are achieved.

Surgical Aspects for Achieving Predictable Results With the GBR Technique for Ridge Augmentation

1. Use of systematic and meticulous low-trauma surgical technique to minimize insult to the bone and the soft tissue flap

2. Use of a lateral incision technique with a combined split-thickness/full-thickness flap design

3. Use of an appropriate e-PTFE membrane

4. Creation and maintenance of a space underneath the membrane using autogenous corticocancellous bone grafts stabilized with supporting screws

5. Stabilization and close adaptation of the membrane to the surrounding bone with fixation screws

6. Achievement of a primary soft tissue healing

7. Healing period of 9 months

Use of an Appropriate Barrier Membrane

In the presented clinical study, e-PTFE membranes were exclusively used. These membranes were specifically designed for GBR procedures of the alveolar ridge (see Chapter 4). The structure of the inner portion of this membrane does not allow the penetration of cells through the membrane, which is an important factor for successful function as a physical barrier. Histologic analysis in a recently published experimental study by Schenk et al[4] has demonstrated that this membrane material is bioinert, allows a complication-free tissue integration, and functions successfully as a GBR barrier (see Chapter 3). This study confirmed observations in previous histologic studies.[5,6] As an alternative to bioinert membranes, biodegradable membranes have only been tested for periodontal indications in recent years.[7-12]

Membrane Stabilization and Close Adaptation to Surrounding Bone

Close adaptation of the membrane is necessary to achieve a sealing effect, preventing the ingrowth of competing soft tissue cells derived from the overlying mucosa. According to the GBR principle, these cells are able to compete with bone-forming cells in the secluded space underneath the membrane. In addition, stabilization of the membrane is helpful in protecting the blood clot and in maintaining close adaptation of the membrane to the bone surface during wound closure. The specially designed stainless steel fixation screws of the Memfix System facilitate membrane application, adaptation to the surrounding bone, membrane stabilization, and removal during the second-stage surgery.

Creation and Maintenance of a Secluded Space

The complete or partial collapse of the membrane by the soft tissue pressure observed in a few patients in this study caused a reduction of possible gain in crest width. Therefore, an appropriate membrane-supporting device is useful in surgical sites where the GBR technique is used to enlarge the width of the alveolar crest. Collagen Fleece did not provide good membrane support, although this product is an excellent blood clot stabilizer and has been used successfully for the treatment of large cystic lesions.[13] Thus, this inexpensive product has its main indication combined with barrier membranes for infrabony defects. The use of supporting screws of the Memfix System in extended edentulous spaces improved the results; however, partial membrane collapse lateral to the supporting screws still occurred. This problem was ultimately solved with the use of autogenous corticocancellous bone grafts stabilized with supporting screws. These bone grafts were exclusively harvested from donor sites within the oral cavity. The preferred donor site was the retromolar area of the mandible, followed by the chin. These grafts were taken with a cortical portion approximately 2 mm thick and a cancellous inner portion. The grafts were placed with the cancellous portion in contact with the recipient bone surface. In combination with bone grafts, the e-PTFE membrane has a double function: *(1)* it serves as a GBR barrier to allow bone formation in the secluded space underneath the membrane around the applied bone grafts and *(2)* it appears to serve as a graft preservation device, protecting the bone grafts from resorption processes. Furthermore, the combination of barrier membranes with autogenous bone grafts seems to improve the quality of the bone structure, which is advantageous in potential recipient sites for implants with a spongy bone structure, such as the posterior maxilla. The latter two clinical observations have to be confirmed with a large number of patients. In addition, the details of graft integration, graft remodeling, and substitution patterns underneath membranes are not known at present and are under investigation in an ongoing experimental study. Alternatives to autogenous bone grafts, such as hydroxyapatite[14] or demineralized freeze-dried bone grafts,[15] have been discussed in previous chapters.

Achievement of Primary Soft Tissue Healing

The importance of primary soft tissue healing has been demonstrated in this as well as other clinical and experimental studies.[16–19] Primary soft tissue healing depends on the incision technique, flap design, handling of the soft tissues during surgery, postoperative monitoring, and patient compliance. The systematic use of a lateral incision technique (avoiding midcrestal incisions) and appropriate relieving incisions distant from the membrane margins drastically reduced the rate of flap dehiscences in this study. Meticulous soft tissue handling using especially fine instruments to minimize the trauma to the combined split-thickness/full-thickness flap was considered to be a key factor. With this flap design, superficial necrosis of the epithelial layer at the tip of the flap was frequently seen. However, this had no negative influence on the soft tissue healing, since the connective tissue maintained its vitality and healed by concentric re-epithelization. The healing process appeared to be accelerated by the frequent application of Solcoseryl dental adhesive paste.

Postoperative Recommendations
1. Perioperative antibiotic coverage with amoxycillin (750 mg 3 to 4 times per day) for 2 to 3 days
2. Perioperative medication with a non-steroidal anti-inflammatory (diclofenac 50 mg tid for 3 days)
3. Application of a tight extraoral elastoplast pressure dressing for 3 days
4. Extraoral application of cold packs in the treated area
5. Local application of Solcoseryl dental adhesive paste to accelerate soft tissue healing (3 times daily for 2 to 3 weeks)
6. Hollowing out of existing provisional partial dentures to avoid direct contact with the wound bed
7. Chemical plaque control for 2 to 3 weeks

Sufficient Healing Period

As already mentioned at the beginning of this chapter, the staged approach for localized ridge augmentation is utilized in patients with more extended bone defects. As a consequence, bone formation and bone maturation need more time in these larger defects when compared to the smaller defects treated with the simultaneous approach. A relatively long healing period was used in this clinical study, since the newly formed alveolar ridge must sustain the surgical trauma during the second-stage surgery for the placement of endosseous implants. Since the details of time sequence of bone remodeling in membrane-protected bone defects are not known at present, the conservative recommendation of 9 months of healing offers less risk for the patient. Future research will demonstrate if the recommended healing period can be shortened.

Summary

After a development period of 3 years, the described GBR technique can be considered a clinically approved procedure for localized ridge augmentation. If the presented surgical technique is followed, a successful result can be achieved with a predictability of more than 90%. However, the technique is only approved for lateral ridge augmentation in partially edentulous patients. Future clinical research will show if the same technique can also be used for vertical ridge augmentation and for fully edentulous patients. However, the technique will have some limitations imposed by the amount of bone grafts available from the oral cavity. In patients with extremely atrophied, fully edentulous jaws, the use of autogenous bone grafts from the iliac crest with or without barrier membranes is the treatment of choice if endosseous implants are to be inserted (see Chapter 8).

Acknowledgments

The authors thank Mrs Oedipe for drawing the schematic diagrams. The professional assistance of Mrs Gaby Leuenberger and the entire surgical staff at the Department of Oral Surgery, University of Berne, during the surgical procedures in the past 5 years is also greatly appreciated.

References

1. Buser D, Brägger U, Lang NP, Nyman S. Regeneration and enlargement of jaw bone using guided tissue regeneration. Clin Oral Impl Res 1990;1:22.

2. Buser D, Dula K, Belser U, Hirt HP, Berthold H. Localized ridge augmentation using guided bone regeneration. I. Surgical procedure in the maxilla. Int J Periodont Rest Dent 1993;13:29.

3. Buser D, Dula K, Belser U, Hirt HP, Berthold H. Localized ridge augmentation using guided bone regeneration. II. Surgical procedure in the mandible. Int J Periodont Rest Dent (submitted).

4. Schenk RK, Buser D, Hardwick WR, Dahlin C. Healing pattern of bone regeneration in membrane-protected defects. A histologic study in the canine mandible. Int J Oral Maxillofac Implants 1994;9:13–29.

5. Dahlin C, Linde A, Gottlow J, Nyman S. Healing of bone defects by guided tissue regeneration. Plast Reconstr Surg 1988;81:672.

6. Dahlin C, Gottlow J, Linde A, Nyman S. Healing of maxillary and mandibular bone defects using a membrane technique. Scand J Plast Reconstr Hand Surg 1990;24:13.

7. Magnusson I, Batich C, Collins BR. New attachment formation following controlled tissue regeneration using biodegradable membranes. J Periodontol 1988;59:1.

8. Fleisher N, De Waal H, Bloom A. Regeneration of lost attachment in the dog using Vicryl absorbable mesh (polyglactin 910). Int J Periodont Rest Dent 1988;8(2):45.

9. Chung KM, Salkin LM, Stein MD, Freedman A. Clinical evaluation of a biodegradable collagen membrane in guided tissue regeneration. J Periodontol 1990;61:732.

10. Schultz AJ, Gager AH. Guided tissue regeneration using absorbable membrane (polyglactin 910) and osseous grafting. Int J Periodont Rest Dent 1990;10:8.

11. Zappa U. Resorbierbare Membranen (I). Parodontale Gewebe-regeneration unter Verwendung von resorbierbaren Membranen—klinische Aspekte. Schweiz Monatsschr Zahnmed 1991;101:1147.

12. Zappa U. Resorbierbare Membranen (II). Parodontale Gewebe-regeneration unter Verwendung von resorbierbaren Membranen—Histologische Aspekte. Schweiz Monatsschr Zahnmed 1991;101:1321.

13. Buser D, Berthold H. Knochendefektfüllung im Kieferbereich mit Kollagenvlies. Dtsch Z Mund Kiefer Gesicht Chir 1986;10:191.

14. Wachtel HC, Langford A, Bernimoulin JP, Reichart P. Guided bone regeneration next to osseointegrated implants in humans. Int J Oral Maxillofac Implants 1991;6:127.

15. Nevins R, Mellonig JT. Enhancement of the damaged edentulous ridge to receive dental implants: A combination of allograft and the GORE-TEX membrane. Int J Periodont Rest Dent 1992;12:97.

16. Jovanovic S, Spiekermann H, Richter EJ. Bone regeneration around titanium dental implants in dehisced defect sites: A clinical study. Int J Oral Maxillofac Implants 1992;7:233.

17. Gotfredsen K, Warrer K, Hjørting-Hansen E, Karring T. Effect of membranes and hydroxyapatite on healing in bone defects around titanium implants. An experimental study in the monkey. Clin Oral Impl Res 1991;2:172.

18. Warrer K, Gotfredsen K, Hjørting-Hansen E, Karring T. Guided tissue regeneration allowing immediate implantation of dental implants into extraction sockets. An experimental study in the monkey. Clin Oral Impl Res 1991;2:166.

19. Gotfredsen K, Nimb L, Buser D, Hjørting-Hansen E. Evaluation of guided bone regeneration around implants placed into fresh extraction sockets. An experimental study in dogs. J Oral Maxillofac Surg 1993;51:879.

CHAPTER EIGHT

Guided Bone Graft Augmentation

Ole T. Jensen

The rationale for bone graft augmentation of the jaws involves not only a biologic basis for graft incorporation but is concerned with graft preservation and adaptability of the graft as it functions in its new environment. Various strategies are used in maxillofacial surgery to promote persistence of the graft: interpositional grafts; the combination of particulate graft with nonresorbable or resorbable hydroxyapatite; the use of metal, alloplast, or allogeneic cribs and bone grafting done in conjunction with osseointegrated implants.[1–8]

To improve the results of these procedures, barrier membranes have been used with the placement of topically applied autografts or allografts over the osseous defects. Early results have demonstrated consistent histologic persistence and viability of the graft.[9–12]

Although guided bone regeneration (GBR) without bone grafting has contributed to clinically successful cases, large defects or augmentations require that graft materials be used. Bone grafts in these settings assume a more prominent role in successful treatment. Bone volume expansions often need to be expanded by a factor of 10 or more for implants to be placed dependably, which is much beyond the capacity of GBR alone.[13,14]

Guided bone graft augmentation (GBGA) designates a barrier membrane application to help preserve and maintain the bone graft itself, and is thus distinguished from GBR where graft material is not used. The use of a membrane to cover a graft in maxillofacial surgery finds its roots in the treatment of jaw continuity defects treated with autogenous grafting, metal cribs, and Millipore filters.[15]

Alveolar augmentation using GBGA introduces a paradigm shift that presages an orthognathic approach to form, function, and esthetics. Implant angulation, position, and stability are enhanced. The load-bearing capacity of the restoration is theoretically increased by permitting an increased number and length of implants. However, for GBGA to be advantageous there must be prudent clinical judgment in treatment planning, primary closure capability using well-vascularized flaps, adequate host healing capacity, and favorable preoperative and postoperative medical and dental management. Successful treatment requires not only proper surgical technique but a treatment protocol that satisfies the biologic constraints of the subperiosteal envelope.

Osseous volume enhancements made to the jaws can be planned using ideal requirements but must take into account the bony base available. In the maxilla there is frequently vertical and horizontal alveolar insufficiency as well as prominent posterior pneumatization. In the mandible the most common defect is posterior horizontal and vertical dimensional insufficiency. Two particular difficulties are also found in the mandible: *(1)* the position of the inferior alveolar nerve within the corpus and *(2)* vertical augmentation limitations imposed by decreased interincisal space. Suggested solutions to these problems have included inferior border augmentation grafting and nerve repositioning surgery.[16–17]

Guided bone graft augmentation in the totally edentulous state must take into account basic treatment plans, available jaw and site bone volumes, and surgical techniques that can achieve stable results long term. Almost all of these procedures will be done with the placement of osseointegrated implants in mind. For this reason, well-integrated 10-mm implant is projected as a minimum treatment goal. The various operations employed are thus designed to create augmented alveoli that can house implants at least 10 mm in length.

Four operative procedures based on the work of Tatum, Breine, Brånemark, and Dahlin[18–25] are modified to take advantage of GBGA:

1. The sinus lift procedure
2. Total lateral alveolar augmentation with or without sinus lift
3. Total vertical alveolar augmentation
4. Nasal floor mucosal lift

Figure 8-1 describes guidelines used in treating patients who have inadequate bone volume for housing an implant of sufficient length. A length of 10 mm is arbitrarily selected as desirable for an implant, and the site classification, for the sake of simplicity, is based on a 10-mm implant. Expanded polytetrafluoroethylene (e-PTFE) is used whenever implant exposure of signifi-

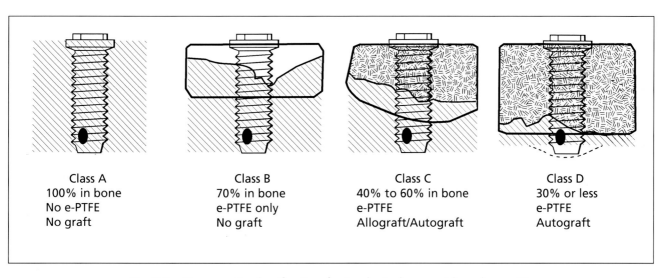

Class A
100% in bone
No e-PTFE
No graft

Class B
70% in bone
e-PTFE only
No graft

Class C
40% to 60% in bone
e-PTFE
Allograft/Autograft

Class D
30% or less
e-PTFE
Autograft

Fig 8-1 Osseous site classification for implant placement based on a 10-mm dental implant. Failure analysis using this system has determined an increased implant failure rate proportional to decreased available basal bone. Grafting has been shown to increase longevity of the Class C and D sites.

cance is present. In general, bone grafting is avoided unless 30% of the implant is exposed at the time of initial placement, because e-PTFE used alone will lead to more intimate bony contact along the surface of the implant than will grafting. However, allografts and autografts are used if about half of the implant is exposed and can be stabilized adequately in basal bone. Autografts, most often obtained from the iliac crest, are used in Class D situations where 30% or less of the implant is secured in basal bone.[25]

A Class A implant that is greater than 10 mm in length but still showing dehiscence facially is frequently grafted and treated with e-PTFE for periodontal or esthetic reasons. The guidelines suggested in Fig 8-1 are based on the clinical impression that load-bearing capacity of the implant is improved by grafting. However, this clinical empiricism is based on improved implant survival and not yet on quantitative loading research.[18–22]

It is hoped that experimental animal studies in the future will refine and demarcate this clinically based protocol with definitive threshold loading data to establish a biomechanical delineation. At present, reliance on current bone loading theory, such as the Carter hypothesis, is helpful when considering the special case of dental implant loading in grafted bone.[26]

The Carter Hypothesis

Applying Carter's bone loading theory to the bone grafting situation, where transosseous titanium implants are placed in sinus or alveolar augmentation bone graft, is derivative of studies and concepts based on the function of mature lamellar bone. Whether titanium implants function the same way in grafted or ungrafted bone is not known, but the basic principle of bone grafting is to attempt to create load-bearing lamellar bone.

In bone grafting of the maxillary sinus, for example, most sterile spacemaking materials, including blood clots, alloplasts, allografts, and autografts, have been shown to form bone. It is not known whether these various grafts respond like cancellous maxillary bone (ie, being anisotropic, adaptable, and fully vital as adjacent basal bone), which may be important in the maintenance of osseointegration.[27-33]

Cortical bone, such as that found in the mandible, has a 50% greater turnover rate when dental implants are present compared to the normal setting. This may be due to a repair stimulus caused by compressive and tensile loading damage adjacent to the implants. As bone fatigue microdamage accumulates during masticatory function, an increased bone turnover rate acts to repair or maintain the structural integrity of osseointegration. The remodeling effect of newly grafted bone in these settings is even more pronounced.[34]

According to the Carter hypothesis, the relationship between bone strain and the net rate of bone volume change in mature bone is a linear function that describes the remodeling response of cortical bone to mechanical loading (Fig 8-2). At high strain rates (3,000 microstrain), a hypertrophic response develops. Conversely, microstrains below 2,000 lead to calcium loss and bone atrophy. Stresses of 4,000 microstrain cause site-specific microdamage exceeding the mechanical threshold of bone in as few as 5,000 cycles. The accumulated bone strain quickly reaches the "fatigue life" of the bone, and fatigue fracture occurs. Frost has termed this the microdamage threshold, which for osseointegrated implants is manifest in mandibular stress fractures or implant and osseous tissue loss due to overloading.[35-39]

The titanium-bone interface of loaded dental implants as measured by radiodensitometry demonstrates a hypertrophic response, ie, increased mineralization next to the implant. This is true for both maxillary and mandibular bone, which have been shown to require increased torque removal force to dislodge implants with time in function. This implies, according to the hypothesis, that a vital reparative remodeling response is taking place next to the dental implant and that it is directly related to the functional state of the implant. A hypertrophic response has also been reported vertically around individual implants and at distant sites such as in the

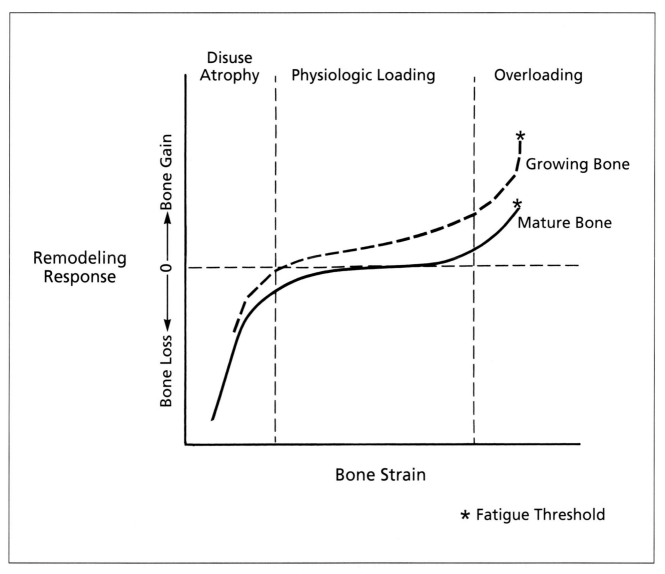

Fig 8-2 Derived from the Carter hypothesis on the relationship between bone strain and cortical bone volume change, fixed titanium implants are theorized to have a remodeling response in direct relationship to the bone strain caused by the implant in function. Fatigue threshold *(asterisk)* is reached earlier in mature bone than in growing bone. Favorable loading of a grafted implant would ideally parallel this mathematic function.[37]

posterior mandible treated with anterior implants only. This hypertrophic response appears to be related to stress imposed by the implant to the bone, especially at the cervical margin, and is not present in unloaded, nonfunctional, or poorly integrated implants.[40–46]

The question then arises, given the dynamics of osseointegration: *What is the best bone grafting material and/or best bone grafting technique to use when titanium implants are planned?* A Wolffian correlate might state that a bone graft must remodel like basal bone in response to the stress and strain of its new environment, otherwise osseointegration is compromised.

The difficulty of achieving this type of bone response in the grafted area is evident by the historically poor performance of corticocancellous block grafts used to treat continuity defects of the mandible. Similarly, corticocancellous grafts combined with dental implants have shown a much higher rate of implant loss and have been reported to have a bone loss rate of up to 2 mm or more per year over the first 2 years after grafting.[22,47,48]

These clinical results are likely related to the grafted cortical bone being largely nonvital and unable to respond adequately to function (ie, microdamage insults) until it is fully resorbed and replaced. Most cortical grafts, however, are never fully resorbed but remain admixtures of dead bone despite developing net bone strengths equal to adjacent nongrafted areas. Whether the devitalized bone could lead to loss of osseointegration is uncertain, but this possibility has been suggested by Roberts et al.[49] Alloplast has also been shown not to contribute significantly to cervical bone formation and maintenance.[50]

Carter et al[36,37] have shown that compressive microdamage results from oblique fractures that run through cellular lacunae and canaliculi, stimulating an extensive cellular response to repair. Repair capability is impaired in devitalized bone or alloplast combined grafts. This mechanism may help to explain findings reported by Roberts et al[49] that early loading of dental implants led to remodeling of devitalized bone, undermining the periosteal margin integrity of titanium implants.

If devitalized bone can affect osseointegration in the nongraft situation, this issue requires even more attention in the grafted situation where most or all of the bone graft material is nonvital.

Maxillofacial bone grafting is therefore accomplished with the end goal of producing a dynamic osseous bed capable of maintaining osseointegration repair. Bone grafting strategies must be well grounded in basic science, leading to bone graft incorporation that is not just prosthetically load bearing but capable of responding anabolically to function over time.

With this theoretical construct in mind, four basic tenets of guided bone graft augmentation are proposed:

1. Use of bone graft material that will be entirely resorbed and replaced as vital bone.

2. Use of a graft stabilization strategy that avoids micromotion or early loading.
3. Use of a barrier membrane to assist in graft preservation and improve contiguity to basal bone.
4. Placement of titanium implants following graft maturation.

Bone Graft Material

The use of cancellous bone is favored over cortical bone for several reasons. In cancellous bone grafts, revascularization is rapid and, therefore, likely to preserve osteogenic cells. Cancellous graft repair is initiated by osteoblasts and is primarily appositional to the existing trabecular framework. New bone is annealed to central cores of dead bone, which are subsequently resorbed and entirely replaced by the process of creeping substitution.[52-54]

Conversely, the cortical bone graft is slowly revascularized. The initial response is osteoclastic, featuring early osteogenic cell death and late vascular anastomosis. Animal studies show a continuous increase in the rate of resorption during the first year after grafting with cortical bone. When cortical bone begins the apposition phase (12 weeks in the dog), the new bone that is formed seals off necrotic bone. Cortical grafts never completely repair but remain an admixture of necrotic bone for years after grafting. This experimental finding appears to be consistent with the clinical incidence of human long bone fractures that most often occur 6 to 18 months after segmental cortical grafting.[55-60]

Because of these laboratory and clinical orthopedic results, and the poor experience maxillofacial surgeons have had using cortical block grafts in the mandible to treat discontinuity defects, efforts to use more viable cancellous grafts (usually from the iliac crest) have gained favor.[61,62]

Graft Stabilization and Preservation

When particulate graft is employed alone, stabilization of the graft is impossible without a crib or a fixation device. Allogeneic or titanium cribs have been used, but inner table iliac grafts will yield a highly flexible continuous graft with 1 mm or less of cortical bone component that can be fixed to the residual jaws by various means.[63,64]

Orthopedic bone screws, plates, or screw-form titanium implants can be used for rigid fixation of the graft. When dental implants are used in highly resorbed areas such as the maxilla, their subsequent use as dental prosthetic abutments is doubtful

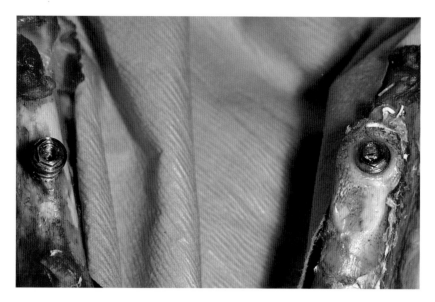

Fig 8-3 Mandible of a foxhound 6 months after grafting with implant-stabilized corticocancellous autograft with and without e-PTFE barriers. The implant treated with e-PTFE *(right)* had 100% bone preservation, whereas the implant without the barrier membrane *(left)* lost more than 50% of the bone graft.[70]

and they are frequently lost because of early loading failure. This is most likely due to poor osseointegration. Submucosal loading and therefore micromotion of the implant under the provisional prosthesis during healing can lead to early loss of supporting bone and implants as well. Therefore, loading is deferred for at least 2 months, ie, no denture prosthesis is worn for that period of time to allow for progress toward consolidation of the graft.[21,22,55]

A cancellous bone graft is extremely vulnerable to early resorption by compressive or tensile loading or fibrous tissue ingrowth, so a barrier membrane is used over the entire cancellous grafted surface laterally. Figure 8-3 shows the results of a 6-month study done in foxhounds, where a corticocancellous graft fixed by an implant was treated with and without e-PTFE barriers. Implants treated with e-PTFE had 100% bone preservation, whereas grafted implants treated without e-PTFE lost 50% or more of the bone graft.[64–70]

The wound overlying the graft is meticulously closed in two layers to avoid wound dehiscence. Exclusion of the periosteum and fibrous tissue elements have repeatedly demonstrated graft preservation by what Murray described as a "caging" effect.[64–70]

Graft preservation observed at exposure surgery 6 to 9 months later features minimal loss of osseous volume. Corticalization of the cancellous grafted surface occurs as early as 4 to 6 months after autogenous grafting and 6 to 12 months after mineralized allogeneic cancellous grafting.[63]

Delayed Implant Placement

Whether implants should be placed at the same time as grafting is controversial. Osseointegration at the light microscopic level is not demonstrable in 1-mm titanium test implants placed immediately into grafted bone sites and later retrieved with a trephine drill at the exposure appointment. A patchy osseointegration is always present despite clinically firm fixation of the implant. Growth factors OP1, PDGF, and IGF-1 placed next to titanium implants have demonstrated osseointegration but are not yet available for clinical use.[71,72]

Carlsson et al[73] showed that osseointegration does not occur unless the osseous gap between titanium and the bony surface is less than about 0.2 mm. Except through the cortical portion of the graft, this close proximity is doubtful in bone graft cases. If function of the cortical portion of the graft leads to resorption, the remaining osseointegration content in the cancellous portion may be inadequate for loading.[73]

Because of this problem, implant longevity in the grafted case is often proportional to the amount of basal bone that is present, especially if there is cortical basal bone present. This is consistent with animal research that has shown that it is the cortical and not the cancellous bone that plays the major role in the torque removal force required to remove an implant.[74] In situations where there is little available basal cortex, the immature graft becomes highly vulnerable to mechanical loading because the cortex is slow in developing. The cancellous graft after 6 to 9 months of healing has less than 2 mm of surface cortex formed. This has led to prosthetic strategies to progressively load the bone until it is fully mature and able to respond to occlusal load. Other strategies that are helpful for graft preservation include implant splinting, avoidance of cantilevers, and avoidance of overdenture torquing through the attachment mechanism.[74–76]

If the bone graft is placed and left to mature for several months prior to placing implants, the implant survival rate increases and implants are more likely to be osseointegrated because much of the bony resorption has already occurred. Also, assuming the graft is viable, greater bone contact will be present and the osseointegration content will be improved. For these reasons, dental implants that must rely on the bone graft for structural support should, when possible, be placed following bone graft maturation until growth factors become available for clinical use.

Sinus Bone Graft Augmentation

Bone grafting of the maxillary sinus is done through a Caldwell-luc or palatal approach. The sinus membrane is lifted with the ostectomized lateral maxillary plate of bone attached to it to limit the created "sub-antral" defect superiority. Cancellous particulate bone graft is packed into the sinus. The graft is then covered laterally by e-PTFE and re-entered 4 to 9 months later for placement of implants. If there is sufficient bone for implant stabilization, implants are placed at the time of grafting.[32]

Examples of GBGA in the sinus illustrate common clinical and histologic features. The sinus bone graft (Figs 8-4 to 8-8) at the stage 2 uncovering 6 to 9 months after grafting almost always is observed to have a caging effect, corticalization of the surface, contiguous graft incorporation, and accentuated vascularity. However, if implants are placed at the time of grafting, there is usually patchy osseointegration (Figs 8-9 and 8-10). These findings, in conjunction with developmental experiences defining the limits of GBGA for the sinus, have led to treatment recommendations in regard to implant placement at the time of bone grafting, as outlined in Table 8-1 and illustrated in Fig 8-11.[32,63,78]

Bone quality is also an important factor in classifying an implant site. If the bone quality is poor, fixation of the implant is not possible despite adequate bone volume.[25,77]

The recommendations in Table 8-1 and Fig. 8-11 are based on clinical experience where the most frequently used sinus bone graft materials are mineralized allogeneic cancellous chips and iliac particulate autograft. The larger the defect, the more likely autogenous grafting will be used. Other sources of bone include mandibular, maxillary, and tibial autograft. Data for the use of demineralized freeze-dried bone, hydroxyapatite, and various composite graft combinations have been covered in earlier chapters. The compilation of the most successful regimen used over a 3-year period is delineated in Table 8-2 according to site classification, bone graft material used, and whether implant placement was immediate or delayed.[65]

Tables 8-2 and 8-3 demonstrate that the more bone there was available for placement of implants, the greater the implant survival rates. Implants that are placed in Class D sites have less than 50% survival rate unless combined with corticocancellous bone graft (84% survival rate).

Delaying implant placement improved early implant survival. Overall, the immediately placed implant survival rate was 81% compared to 93% in the delayed implant placement group. It is not known whether this data will stand up over a 5- or 10-year time span, but very few implants are lost after restoration; most failures occur at or near the time of exposure. Failure to osseointegrate is most frequently attributed to inadequate implant fixation or provisional prosthetic overloading of the grafted implant site.

Sinus grafting—Case 1.   *Figs 8-4a to d*

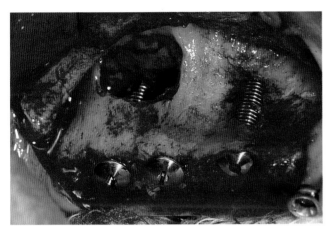

8-4a

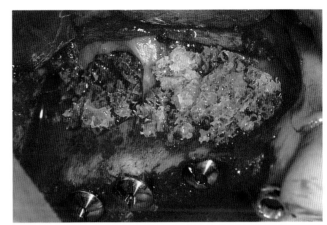

8-4b

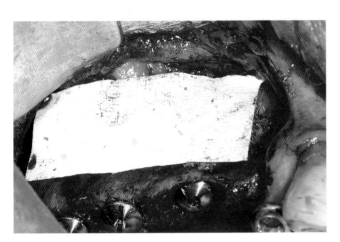

8-4c

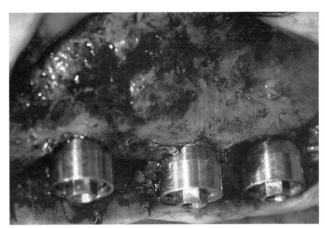

8-4d

Fig 8-4a   Posterior maxilla is pneumatized and narrow, but implant fixation is sufficient to allow immediate placement of implants.

Fig 8-4b   Cancellous bone graft is used to fill the sinus cavity and cover the dehiscence over the anterior implant.

Fig 8-4c   Graft is covered with a barrier membrane.

Fig 8-4d   Six months later, the e-PTFE is removed. The graft is clinically firm.

Sinus grafting—Case 2.   *Figs 8-5a to d*

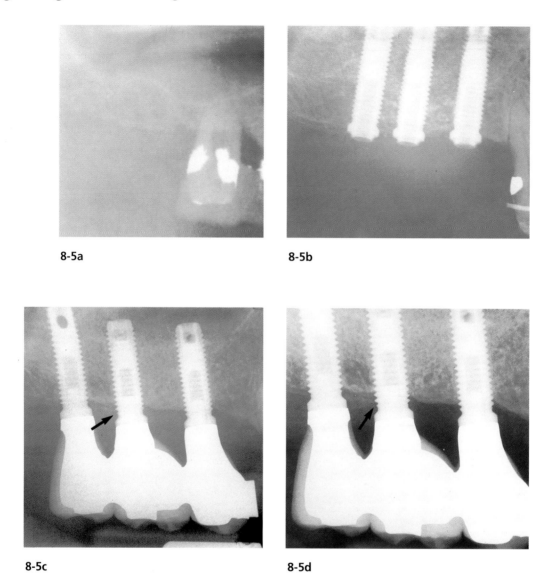

8-5a   8-5b

8-5c   8-5d

Fig 8-5a   Initial loss of alveolar bone in relation to the maxillary sinus.

Fig 8-5b   Three implants are placed with mineralized allogeneic bone graft. The implants are not countersunk to avoid loss of stability.

Fig 8-5c   Nine months later, the implants are exposed and a three-unit fixed prosthesis is constructed (shown here 18 months after implant placement). Note early loss of cortical bone probably due to vascular embarrassment from the surgical procedure *(arrow)*.

Fig 8-5d   At 30 months after graft *(arrow)* is placed, osseous structures appear stable with no further vertical loss of bone.

Sinus grafting—Case 3. *Figs 8-6a to d*

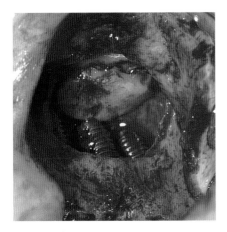

8-6a

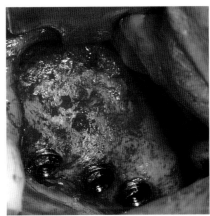

8-6b

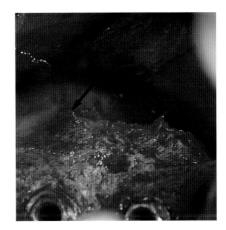

8-6c

Fig 8-6a Sinus cavity is exposed without perforation of the sinus membrane.

Fig 8-6b Six months after grafting, an outpouching of the area grafted under the membrane is observed.

Fig 8-6c Caging effect *(arrows)* of the membrane creates an excess of bone laterally.

Fig 8-6d When a membrane is not used, even when the graft overfills the sinus defect, incleftation and increased scarring is observed.

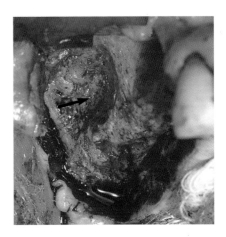

8-6d

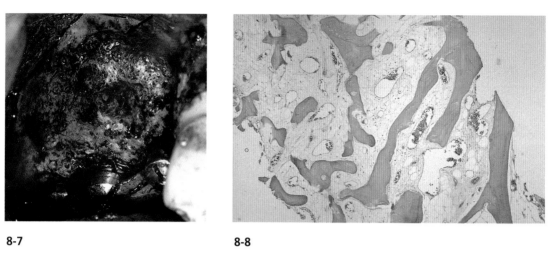

8-7   8-8

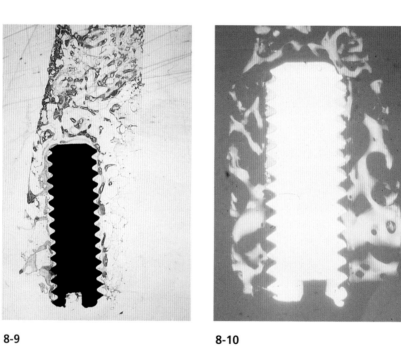

8-9   8-10

Fig 8-7   Margin of the barrier membrane is clearly demarcated by a significant increase in vascularity and corticalization *(arrow)* as part of the caging effect.

Fig 8-8   Biopsy specimen trephined from the antrum in the area of the first molar 6 months after grafting with mineralized allogeneic cancellous chips demonstrates a 15-mm core of highly vascularized vital cancellous bone.

Fig 8-9   A 1-mm titanium bone screw used as a test implant was placed into the sinus graft area at the time of grafting. Six months later, the implant and bone is removed with a trephine, and patchy osseointegration is observed despite the clinically firm appearance of the implant.[78]

Fig 8-10   Microradiography of a retrieved test implant demonstrates vital bone next to less than 25% of the implant in this cancellous bone graft environment.[78]

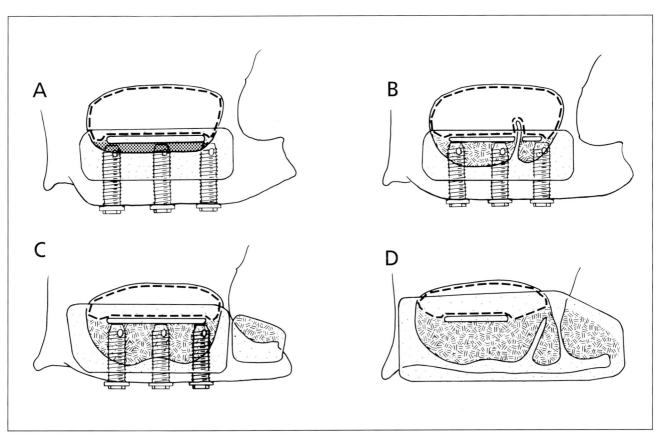

Fig 8-11   This osseous site classification, based on clinical experience, is recommended for most clinical situations. *Class A:* sufficient bone to place at least a 10-mm implant; minor sinus elevation is done to increase implant length; usually no graft material is required, but e-PTFE is used. *Class B:* 7 to 9 mm of available bone; autograft or allograft is used under a barrier membrane and implants are usually placed at the time of grafting. *Class C:* 4 to 6 mm of available bone; autograft or allograft is used with e-PTFE and delayed implant placement. *Class D:* reserved for corticocancellous graft or particulate autograft, e-PTFE, and delayed implant placement; nasal fossa grafting is usually associated with the Class D maxilla.

Table 8-1   *Sinus Bone Graft Classification and Treatment Recommendations*

Site	Graft material	e-PTFE	Implant
Class D (0–3 mm)	Autograft	yes	Delayed
Class C (4–6 mm)	Autograft/Allograft	yes	Delayed or immediate
Class B (7–9 mm)	Autograft/Allograft	yes	Immediate
Class A (10 mm+)	No graft/Blood clot	no	Immediate

Table 8-2 *Implant Survival in Sinus Bone Grafts When Implants Were Placed at the Time of Grafting*

	Class D	Class C	Class B	Class A
Iliac autograft	94/112*	42/51*	14/16	–
Maxillofacial autograft	–	15/18	21/21	–
Tibial autograft	–	4/4	–	–
Mineralized allograft	5/11	53/71	25/28	–

Table 8-3 *Implant Survival in Sinus Bone Grafts When Implants Were Placed 4 to 12 Months After Grafting*

	Class D	Class C	Class B	Class A
Iliac autograft	25/29	13/14	–	–
Maxillofacial autograft	28/31	23/23	14/14	–
Mineralized allograft	–	26/29	26/26	–
Tibial autograft	5/6	–	–	–

Combined Alveolar and Sinus Augmentation

When augmentation grafting is done in conjunction with sinus grafting and immediate or delayed implant placement, early results have demonstrated a much improved graft preservation and longevity when e-PTFE is used. In the 11 patients treated to date with this technique, 11 of 90 implants placed were failures. Seven implant failures occurred in one patient who had no lateral nasal walls and therefore had continuity from the sinus bilaterally with 1 mm or less of vertical alveolar bone available at the time of surgery. Figures 8-12a to l show a series of surgical and restorative findings using a modification of the Brånemark and Breine technique combined with the sinus graft. Facial and lateral corticalization occurred 6 months after grafting despite the use of particulate marrow graft. The final restoration is a fixed removable prosthesis.

Figures 8-13a to h are a series of surgical findings observed in a patient who had multiple maxillary surgeries, including the placement and removal of a subperiosteal implant and multiple attempts at alloplast augmentation with significant morbidity to the patient. These efforts resulted in complete loss of the entire basal alveolus, ablation of the anterior maxilla and anterior palate, and loss of sensory function to the upper lip.

In this type of case, minimal effort is made to secure several implants at the time of grafting because of the compromised tissues. Instead, a few implants or bone plates are used to secure the graft, then implants are placed 6 to 9 months later into well-vascularized and remodeled bone. This enables the placement of implants much more anteriorly and with more confidence that osseointegration will occur. This patient was treated with a spark erosion fixed denture supported by eight osseointegrated implants. Two of four implants used to secure the graft were lost at the time of exposure.

Figures 8-14a to f demonstrate an effort to treat a highly resorbed maxilla with GBGA; greater attention is given to shaping and sculpting of the graft prior to wound closure so that a more ideal form is obtained. This exposure and e-PTFE removal was done 6 months after grafting and demonstrates a highly corticalized and vascularized bone that resembles alveolar form.

Figures 8-15a and b show a biopsy specimen taken 6 months after bone graft surgery. Healthy cancellous bone, taken from the maxillary first molar region, is at least 15 mm in length (the preoperative value was 1 to 2 mm).

Figures 8-16a and b show a composite cephalometric tracing of a patient with radiographs taken preoperatively and 2 and 3 years postsurgery. The implants are 13 to 18 mm in length, with very little change in the overall graft morphology in either jaw over the 3-year period.

Table 8-4 outlines bone volumes found at the time of implant exposure and e-PTFE removal as compared to preoperative levels. The net increase in bone volume is extraordinary when compared to previously used techniques. Total alveolar increases average 11 mm with a range of 8 to 15 mm or more when e-PTFE is used. In most of the sinus graft areas the net increase is well above 15 mm, and in some cases in excess of 25 mm in the first molar areas. Discernible change in grafted sinus floor morphology is not significant up to 3 years after grafting.

An effort to establish ideal alveolar form by delaying completion of implant placement until the exposure appointment is being pursued. The horseshoe-shaped corticocancellous graft may require as few as two implants to adequately stabilize it, followed by the addition of 4 to 6 implants at the exposure appointment. This is particularly helpful in treating patients with retromaxillary positions, or patients who have experienced subperiosteal implant failure or undergone tumor resection, where the final position of the implants is desired to be more anterior than is possible in the initial surgery (Fig 8-17).

The argument for delayed placement of implants is based not only on finding a solution to fixation difficulties but on obtaining increased proximity of the implant to the bone.[73]

Figure 8-18 illustrates recommended treatment for the highly resorbed maxilla when a fixed prosthesis is planned. Note that the severely atrophic and retropositioned maxilla is treated in a delayed fashion, whereas the orthognathic maxilla (Fig 8-19) may be treated with immediate implant placement, but only if the implants can be well stabilized in basal bone.

Modified Brånemark and Breine technique with sinus graft in 50-year-old woman who had worn a complete maxillary denture against dentition for 22 years. *Figs 8-12a to l*

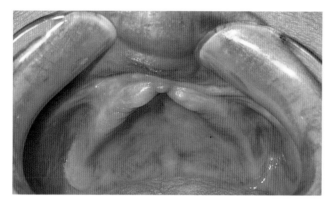

8-12a

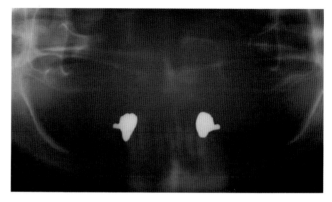

8-12b

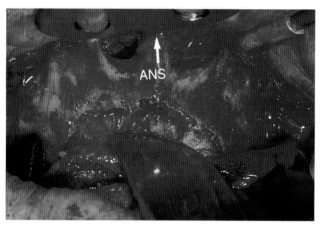

8-12c

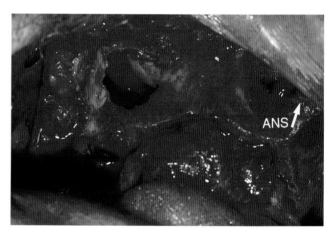

8-12d

Figs 8-12a and b Most alveolar areas have 1 to 2 mm of residual bone remaining.

Figs 8-12c and d Sinus and nasal lifts are performed, preserving the anterior nasal spine (ANS).

Fig 8-12e Palatal mucosa is not reflected *(asterisk)*.

Fig 8-12f Implants extend into the maxillary sinus *(arrow)*.

Fig 8-12g The antrae, nasal fossae, and lateral and anterior maxillae are packed with particulate cancellous marrow from the iliac crest.

Fig 8-12h Barrier membrane covers the entire cancellous graft.

Fig 8-12i Six months after grafting, the implants are exposed and the membrane is removed.

Fig 8-12j Corticalization and graft preservation is observed.

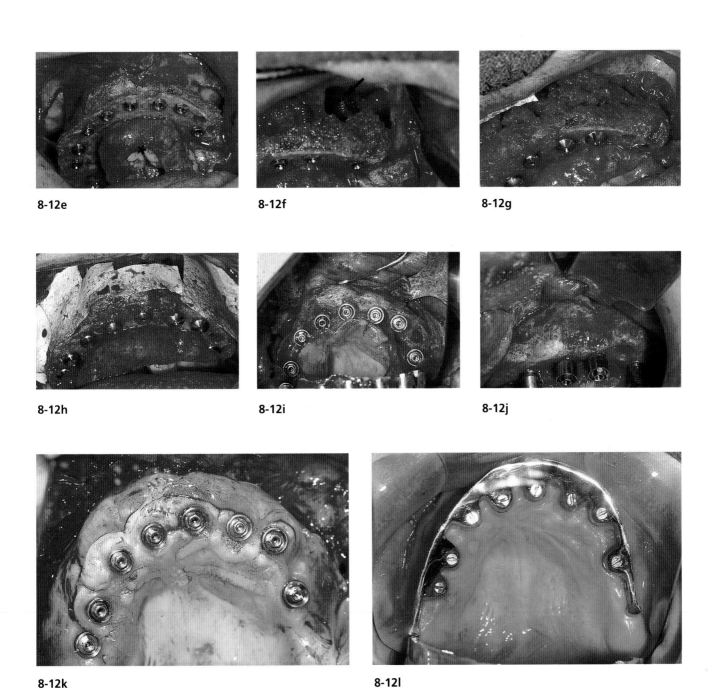

8-12e

8-12f

8-12g

8-12h

8-12i

8-12j

8-12k

8-12l

Fig 8-12k Six weeks later, a modified Edlan flap (lip switch vestibuloplasty) creates a new vestibule.

Fig 8-12l Thirty months after the initial surgery, the implants are stable and the graft is still in place.

Combined grafting of 62-year-old patient who had been in renal failure in the past.   *Figs 8-13a to h*

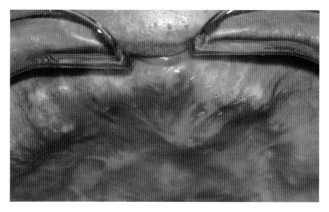

8-13a

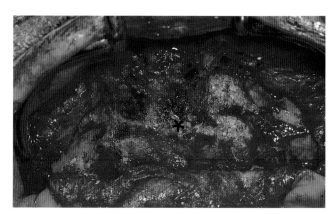

8-13b

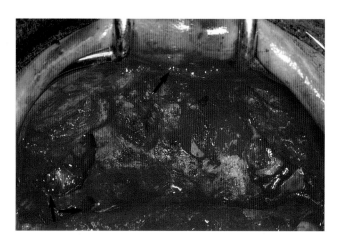

8-13c

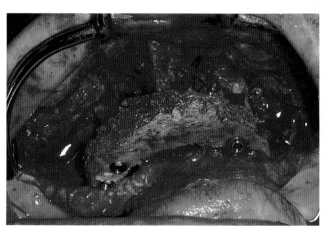

8-13d

Fig 8-13a   Initial treatment with a subperiosteal implant had completely destroyed the basal bone of the maxillary alveolus.

Fig 8-13b   The failing implant also ablated the anterior palate, exposing the nasal fossa into the midpalatal region *(asterisk).*

Fig 8-13c   Anterior nasal spine was absent *(arrow)* and there were areas of dehiscence from the palate *(arrows)* and lateral maxilla that became evident in the process of performing the sinus lift procedure. Alloplast that had been placed in an effort to salvage the implant was also removed.

Fig 8-13d   Four implants are used to secure the corticocancellous graft, as the osseointegration potential is guarded.

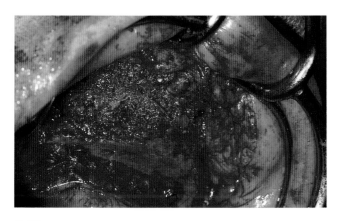

8-13e

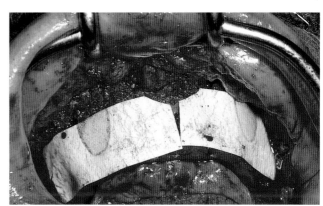

8-13f

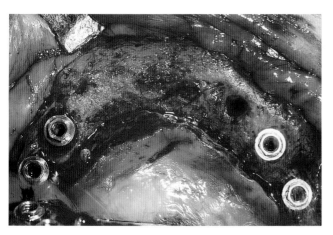

8-13g

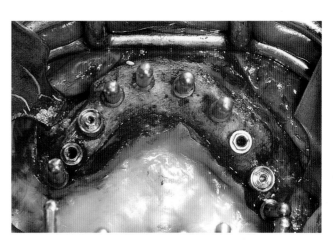

8-13h

Fig 8-13e Since the nasal floor and palate is also reconstructed in this case, marrow graft is packed under the advanced horseshoe-shaped corticocancellous graft.

Fig 8-13f Barrier membrane is placed before the wound is closed with a two-layer technique.

Fig 8-13g Six months after surgery, the graft is exposed. Two of the four fixation implants were lost, whereas none of the delayed-placement implants was lost.

Fig 8-13h Additional implants are placed.

Fig 8-14a Exposure of the graft and implants 7 months after surgery. Implants are 13 to 18 mm in length and are all integrated.

Fig 8-14b More attention is given to the shape of the graft at the time of surgery because so little graft is lost during the incorporation period if the denture is not used for 2 months after surgery.

Fig 8-14c When an e-PTFE membrane extends over the implant head, there is minimal bone loss but increased risk of barrier membrane exposure. The membrane does not cover the entire graft unless two-layer closure is obtainable.

Fig 8-14d Sinus-grafted area at 7 months after grafting illustrates a mottled cortex that can be scratched with an explorer but is still quite thin and immature.

Fig 8-14e Overall shape of the regenerated maxilla at the time of exposure of the implants. The exposure incision is palatal so that keratinized gingiva is transposed buccally.

Fig 8-14f Six weeks later, the vestibuloplasty is done and keratinization is found around most of the implants.

Highly resorbed maxilla (2 to 3 mm of residual bone) of 56-year-old man treated with corticocancellous augmentation and sinus graft with immediate implant placement. *Figs 8-14a to f*

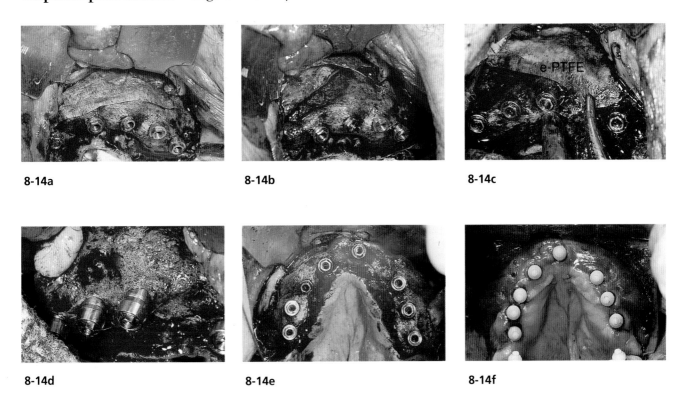

8-14a

8-14b

8-14c

8-14d

8-14e

8-14f

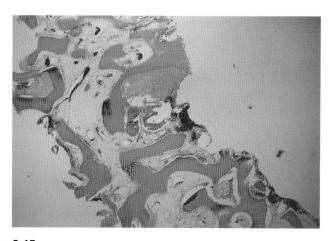

8-15a

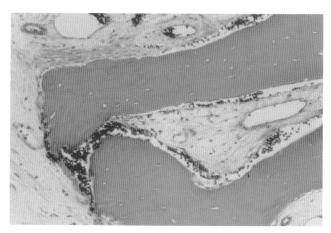

8-15b

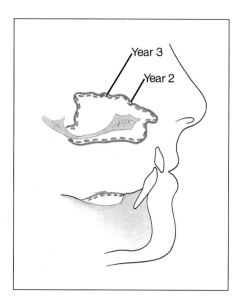

8-16a

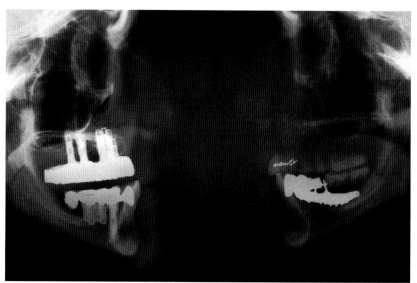

8-16b

Fig 8-15a A trephine biopsy core extending through the alveolus into the grafted maxillary sinus demonstrates a cancellous architecture.

Fig 8-15b At higher power, the bone shows cells within lacunae and osteoblastic activity. This pattern is a consistent finding in more than 30 biopsy samples observed.[65,78]

Figs 8-16a and b Preoperative and postoperative cephalograms demonstrate vertical persistence of the guided bone graft augmentation done in both jaws of a 50-year-old female patient. The preoperative anterior maxilla was absent, with severe Class D sites present in both jaws. The patient was treated with fixed prostheses and had minimal bone loss during the second and third year after grafting.

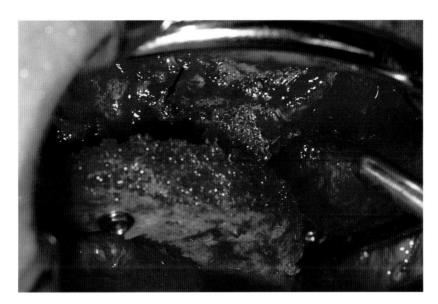

Fig 8-17 Residual alveolus can be advanced up to 15 mm in patients who present with iatrogenic, ablative, or developmental Class II jaw relationships. Arrow shows anterior-most alveolar residuum. Overlying graft advances the maxilla 15 mm.

Table 8-4 *Combined Maxillary Augmentation and Sinus Grafting With Immediate and Delayed Implant Placement in 11 Patients*

Patient	Preoperative average bone volume (mm)‡	Bone volume at exposure of implants (mm)‡	Net increase (mm)
JH*	2	8	6
SH	2	13	11
DS	3	15	12
LL†	1	9	8
ES	1–2	14	12
BA	0–1	15	14
AB	3	14	11
JC	3	15	12
CA	4	15	11
SS	2	13	11
DE	1–2	13	11

*No e-PTFE was used and no sinus graft was done.
†Seven of eight implants did not integrate. There were no lateral nasal walls, and the sinus cavities were contiguous with the nasal fossa. Despite this, bone volume was increased by a factor of nearly 8 times and the implants placed at a later date integrated well.
‡Maxillary bone volume was measured directly at the time of surgery in four positions and then averaged to the nearest millimeter. The measurements are taken at approximately the canine and first molar areas. At present, these surgeries are reserved for patients with 3 mm or less of residual basal bone.

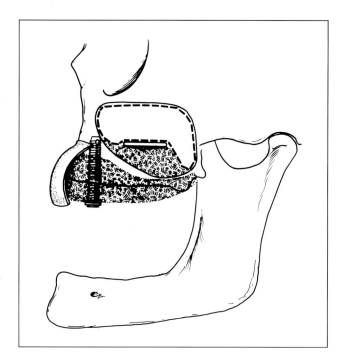

8-18

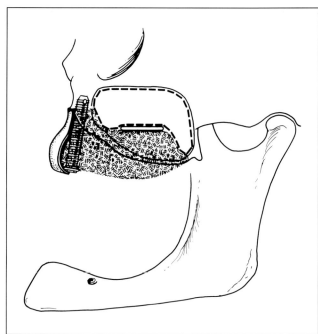

8-19

Fig 8-18 If the jaws are in a Class I relationship, even if very minimal bone is available for securing implants, four to eight implants can usually be placed and expected to integrate.

Fig 8-19 In a severe Class II situation, as few as two implants can be placed and used as fixation devices. When the graft matures, implants that will be more likely to osseointegrate can be placed and used with more confidence in the dental restoration. The problem of difficult implant positioning is also alleviated by using the delayed implant placement approach.

Placement of the graft and subsequent delay of implant placement until the exposure appointment has numerous technical and physiologic advantages that may not be outweighed by the convenience of an aggressive surgery that attempts to accomplish both graft incorporation and osseointegration.

Summary

The use of the barrier membrane as an adjunct to already available surgical grafting techniques advances progress toward complete restoration of alveolar form. Guided bone graft augmentation will likely hold long-term promise as it is refined in preparation for the recombinant products that presumably will need a crib or barrier to establish appropriate local alveolar response.

References

1. Lindstrom J, Brånemark P-I, Albrektsson, T. Mandibular reconstruction using the preformed autologous bone graft. J Plas Reconstr Surg 1981;15:29.

2. Boyne PJ. The use of marrow particulate grafts and titanium implants in the reconstruction of resected mandibles. In: Jacobs JR (ed). Maxillofacial Trauma: An International Perspective. New York: Praeger, 1983:212

3. Serra JM, Paloma V, Mesa F. The vascularized fibula graft in mandibular reconstruction. J Oral Maxillofac Surg 1991;49:244.

4. Kraut RA, Kessler HP, Holmes RE. Quantification of bone in dental implant sites after composite grafting of the mandible: Report of a case. Int J Oral Maxillofac Implants 1989;4:153.

5. Kahnberg KE, Nyström E, Bartholdsson L. Combined use of bone grafts and Brånemark fixtures in the treatment of severely resorbed maxillae. Int J Oral Maxillofac Implants 1989;4:297.

6. Keller EE, Van Roekel NB, Desjardins RP, Tolman DE. Prosthetic-surgical reconstruction of the severely resorbed maxilla with iliac bone grafting and tissue-integrated prostheses. Int J Oral Maxillofac Implants 1987;2:155.

7. Bell WH, Buckles RL. Correction of atrophic alveolar ridge by interpositional bone grafting: A progress report. J Oral Surg 1978;36:693.

8. Kent JN, Quinn JH, Zide MF, Guerra LR, Boyne PJ. Alveolar ridge augmentation using nonresorbable hydroxylapatite with or without autogenous cancellous bone. J Oral Maxillofac Surg 1983;41:629.

9. Anderegg CR, Martin ST, Gray JL. Clinical evaluation of the use of decalcified freeze dried bone allograft with guided tissue regeneration in the treatment of molar furcation invasions. J Periodontol 1991;62:264.

10. Stahl SS, Froums S. Histologic healing response in human vertical lesions following the use of osseous allografts and barrier membranes. J Clin Periodontol 1991;18:145.

11. Seibert J, Nyman S. Localized ridge augmentation in dogs: A pilot study using membranes and hydroxylapatite. J Periodontol 1990;61:157.

12. Becker W, Becker B, Handelsman M, Ochsenbein C, Albrektsson T. Guided tissue regeneration for implants placed into extraction sockets: A study in dogs. J Periodontol 1991;62:703.

13. Arora BK, Worley M, Guttu RL, Laskin DM. Bone formation over partially exposed implants using guided tissue regeneration. J Oral Maxillofac Surg 1992;50:1060.

14. Schmid J, Haemmerle HF, Stich H, Lang NP. Supraplant, a novel implant system based on the principle of guided bone generation: A preliminary study in the rabbit. Clin Oral Impl Res 1991;2:199.

15. Boyne PJ. Restoration of osseous defects in maxillofacial casualties. J Am Dent Assoc 1969;78:767.

16. Sanders B. Rib grafting to the inferior border of the mandible. J Oral Surg 1978;36:699.

17. Jensen OT, Nock D. Inferior alveolar nerve repositioning in conjunction with placement of osseointegrated implants: A case report. Oral Surg Oral Med Oral Pathol 1987;63:263.

18. Dahlin C, Sennerby L, Lekholm U, Linde A, Nyman S. Generation of new bone around titanium implants using a membrane technique: An experimental study in rabbits. Int J Oral Maxillofac Implants 1989;4:19.

19. Adell R, Lekholm U, Gröndahl K, Brånemark P-I, Lindström J, Jacobsson M. Reconstruction of severely resorbed edentulous maxillae using osseointegrated fixtures in immediate autogenous bone grafts. Int J Oral Maxillofac Implants 1990; 5:233.

20. Lindstrom RD, Symington JM. Osseointegrated dental implants in conjunction with bone grafts. Int J Oral Maxillofac Implants 1988;3:31.

21. Tolman DE, Desjardins RP, Keller EE. Surgical-prosthodontic reconstruction of oral nasal defects utilizing the tissue-integrated prosthesis. Int J Oral Maxillofac Implants 1988;3:31.

22. Jensen J, Sindet-Pedersen S. Autogenous mandibular bone grafts and osseointegrated implants for reconstruction of the severely atrophic maxilla: A preliminary report. J Oral Maxillofac Surg 1991;49:1277.

23. Breine U, Brånemark P-I. Reconstruction of alveolar jaw bone. An experimental and clinical study of immediate and preformed autologous bone grafts in combination with osseointegrated implants. Scand J Plast Reconstr Surg 1980;4:23.

24. Higuchi KW. Nasal inlay bone graft technique. In: Laney WR, Tolman DE (eds). Tissue Integration in Oral, Orthopedic, and Maxillofacial Reconstruction. Chicago: Quintessence, 1992:318-320.

25. Jensen OT. Site selection for the osseointegrated implant. J Prosthet Dent 1989;4:19.

26. Carter DR. Mechanical loading histories and cortical bone remodeling. Calcif Tissue Int 1984;36:S19.

27. Boyne PJ, James RA. Grafting of the maxillary sinus floor with autogenous marrow and bone. J Oral Surg 1980;38:613.

28. Kent JN, Block MS. Simultaneous maxillary sinus floor bone grafting and placement of hydroxylapatite coated implants. J Oral Maxillofac Surg 1989;47:238.

29. Wood RM, Moore DL. Grafting of the maxillary sinus with intraorally harvested autogenous bone prior to implant placement. Int J Oral Maxillofac Implants 1988;3:209.

30. Smiler D, Holmes RE. Sinus lift procedure using hydroxylapatite: A preliminary report. J Oral Implantol 1989;23:239.

31. Whitker JM, James RA, Lozoda J, Cordova C, GaRey DJ. Histological response and clinical evaluation of heterograft and allograft materials in the elevation of the maxillary sinus for the preparation of endosteal dental implant sites. Simultaneous sinus elevation and root form implantation. An eight month autopsy report. J Oral Implantol 1989;15:141.

32. Jensen OT, Perkins S, Van DeWater FW. Nasal fossa and maxillary sinus grafting of implants from a palatal approach. Report of a case. J Oral Maxillofac Surg 1992;50:415.

33. Tatum H. Maxillary sinus implant reconstruction. Dent Clin North Am 1986; 30:207.

34. Roberts WE, Turley PK, Brezniak N, Felder PJ: Bone physiology and metabolism. J Calif Dent Assoc 1987;15(10)54:61.

35. Taylor TD. Osteogenesis of the mandible associated with implant reconstruction: A patient report. Int J Oral Maxillofac Implants 1989;4:227.

36. Carter DR, Caler WE, Spengler DM, Frankel VH. Fatigue behavior of adult cortical bone—the influence of mean strain and strain range. Acta Orthop Scand 1981;52:481.

37. Carter DR, Caler WE. Cycle dependent and time dependent bone fracture with repeated loading. J Biomech Eng 1983;105:166.

38. Frost HM. Transient-steady state phenomena in microdamage physiology: A prosposed algorithm for lamellar bone. Calcif Tissue Int 1989;44:367.

39. Frost HM. Some ABC's of skeletal pathophysiology: 5. Microdamage physiology. Calcif Tissue Int 1991;49:229.

40. Strid KG. Radiographic results: Radiographic procedures. In: Brånemark P-I, Zarb GA, Albrektsson T (eds). Tissue-Integrated Prostheses: Osseointegration in Clinical Dentistry. Chicago: Quintessence, 1985:187-198, 317-327.

41. Hobkirk JA, Schwab J. Mandibular deformation in subjects with osseointegrated implants. Int J Oral Maxillofac Implants 1991;6:319.

42. Shonberg DC, Stith HD, Jameson LM, Chai JY. Mandibular fracture through an endosseous implant. Int J Oral Maxillofac Implants 1992:7:401.

43. Clelland NL, Ismail YH, Zaki HS, Pipko D. Three-dimensional finite element stress analysis in and around the Screw-vent implant. Int J Oral Maxillofac Implants 1991;6:391.

44. Yamanaka E, Tjellstrom A, Jacobsson M, Albrektsson T. Long-term observation on removal torque of directly bone-anchored implants in man. Int J Oral Maxillofac Implants (in press).

45. Arvidson K, Bystedt H, Frykholm A, von Konow L, Lothigius E. A 3-year clinical study of Astra dental implants in the treatment of edentulous mandibles. Int J Oral Maxillofac Implants 1992;7:321.

46. Oikarinen VJ, Siirila HS. Reparative bone growth in an extremely atrophied edentulous mandible stimulated by an osseointegrated implant-supported fixed prosthesis: A case report. Int J Oral Maxillofac Implants 1992;7:541.

47. Kudo D, Fujioka Y. Review of bone grafting for reconstruction of discontinuity defects of the mandible. J Oral Surg 1978;36:791.

48. Lawson W, Biller HF. Mandibular reconstruction: Bone graft techniques. Otolaryngol Head Neck Surg 1987;90:589.

49. Roberts W, Garreto LP, Decastro RA. Remodeling of devitalized bone threatens periosteal margin integrity of endosseous titanium implants with threaded or smooth surfaces: Indications for provisional loading and axially directed occlusion. J Ind Dent Assoc 1989 (Aug/Sept):2.

50. Donohue WB, Macres C. Effect of hydroxylapatite on bone formation around exposed head of titanium implants. J Oral Maxillofac Surg 1990;48:1196.

51. Roberts WE. Bone tissue interface. J Dent Educ 1988;52:805-809.

52. Heiple K, Goldberg VM, Powell AE, Bos GD, Zika OM. Biology of cancellous bone grafts. Orthoped Clin North Am 1987;18(2):179.

53. Urist M, McLean FC. Osteogenic potency and new bone formation by induction in the transplants to the anterior chamber of the eye. J Bone Joint Surg 1952;34A:443.

54. Zeiss IM, Nishet NM, Helsop BF. Studies of transference of bone II vascularization of autologous and homologous implants of cortical bone in rats. Exp Pathol 1960;41:345.

55. Plenk H, Donhel-Mayerhauser M, Matejka M, Watzek G. Experimental comparison of Brånemark and Lederman-type titanium dental screw implants in sheep [abstract]. Abstracts of the World Congress on Implant Biomaterials, Brussels, Belgium.

56. Burchardt H. The biology of bone graft repair. Clin Orthop Rel Res 1983; 1174:31.

57. Burchardt H. Biology of bone transplantation. Orthop Clin North Am 1987; 18(2):187.

58. Enneking WF, Burchardt H. Physical and biological aspects of repair of dog cortical bone transplants. J Bone Joint Surg 1975;57A:232.

59. Ray RD. Vascularization of bone grafts and implants. Clin Orthop 1972;87:43.

60. Abbott LC, Schottstaedt ER, Saunders JB. The evaluation of cortical and cancellous bone as grafting material: A clinical and experimental study. J Bone Joint Surg 1947;29:381.

61. Chen C, Wu T. Reconstruction of mandibular defects with composite autologous iliac bone and freeze-treated allogeneic rib grafts. J Oral Maxillofac Surg 1982;40:29.

62. Spiessel B. A new method of anatomical reconstruction of expansive defects of the mandible with autogenous cancellous bone. J Maxillofac Surg 1980;8:78.

63. Male AJ, Gasser J, Fonseca RJ, Nelson J. Comparison of onlay autologous and allogeneic bone grafts to the maxilla in primates. J Oral Maxillofac Surg 1983;42:487.

64. Boyne PJ. Advances in preprosthetic surgery and implantation. Curr Opin Dent 1991;1:277.

65. Jensen OT, Greer RO. Immediate placement of osseointegrating implants into the maxillary sinus augmented with mineralized cancellous allograft and Gore-Tex: Second stage surgical and histological findings. In: Laney WR, Tolman DE (eds). Tissue Integration in Oral, Orthopedic, and Maxillofacial Reconstruction. Chicago: Quintessence, 1991:321-333.

66. Murray G, Holden R, Roachlau W. Experimental and clinical study of new growth of bone in a cavity. Am J Surg 1951;93:385.

67. Nyman S, Lindhe J, Karring T, Rylander H. New attachment following surgical treatment of human periodontal disease. J Clin Periodontol 1982;9:290.

68. Gottlow J, Nyman S, Lindhe J, Karring T, Wennstrom J. New attachment formation in the human periodontium by guided tissue regeneration: Case reports. J Periodontol 1986;13:604.

69. Jovanovic SA, Spiekermann H, Richter EJ. Bone regeneration around titanium dental implants in dehised defect sites. A clinical study. Int J Oral Maxillofac Implants 1992;7:233.

70. Jensen OT, Greer RO, Johnson L, Kassebaum D. Vertical mandibular augmentation grafting of high profile titanium implants (in preparation).

71. Lynch S, Buser D, Hernandez R, Weber H, Stich H, Fox C, Williams R. Effects of the platelet derived growth factor/insulin like growth factor I combination on bone regeneration around titanium dental implants. J Periodontol 1991;62:710.

72. Rutherford RB, Sampath TK, Rueger DC, Taylor TD. Use of bovine osteogenic protein to promote rapid osseointegration of endosseous dental implants. Int J Oral Maxillofac Implants 1992;7:297.

73. Carlsson L, Rostlund T, Albrektsson B, Albrektsson T. Implant fixation improved by close fit. Cylindrical implant-bone interface studied in rabbits. Acta Orthop Scand 1988;59:272.

74. Sennerby L, Thompson P. The role of insertion site and inflammation of the integration of pure titanium implants. In: Laney WR, Tolman DE (eds). Tissue Integration in Oral, Orthopedic, and Maxillofacial Reconstruction. Chicago: Quintessence, 1990:334.

75. Johansson C, Albrektsson T. Integration of screw implants in the rabbit: A 1-yr follow-up of removal torque of titanium implants. Int J Oral Maxillofac Implants 1987;2:69.

76. Brownd CL. Resilient ball and socket attachment design for the implant overdenture prostheses. In: Laney WR, Tolman DE (eds). Tissue Integration in Oral, Orthopedic, and Maxillofacial Reconstruction. Chicago: Quintessence, 1990:374.

77. Lekholm U, Zarb GA. Patient selection and preparation. In: Brånemark P-I, Zarb GA, Albrektsson T (eds). Osseointegration in Clinical Dentistry. Chicago: Quintessence, 1985:199-204.

78. Jensen OT, Sennerby L. Osseointegration of titanium test implants in maxillary sinus bone graft (in preparation).

Index